Onward!
Navigating Hip Dysplasia,
PAO Surgery, and Beyond

The PAO Project Series

Volume 1

Onward!
Navigating Hip Dysplasia, PAO Surgery, and Beyond

Edited by Jennifer Lesea-Ames

Editors and Proofreaders
Karen Sudre
Jessica Dyke
Erika M. Schreck

Book Design: Jen Lesea-Ames and Erika M. Schreck
Editing and Proofreading: Karen Sudre, Jessica Dyke and Erika M. Schreck
Cover Design: Erika M. Schreck; Cover Photo: Joy Sherlock

Jennifer Lesea-Ames and most contributors in this book are not medical doctors. This book is not intended as a substitute for the medical advice or treatment from a physician. The reader should regularly consult a physician in matters relating to his/her health and particularly with respect to any symptoms that may require diagnosis or medical attention. The intent of the author is only to offer information of a general nature to help the reader in his/her quest for support and well-being. In the event the reader uses any of the information in this book, which is his/her constitutional and individual right, the author and the publisher assume no responsibility for the reader's actions or results.

Printed in the USA.

Library of Congress Cataloging-in-Publication Data
Lesea-Ames, Jennifer
  Onward! navigating hip dysplasia, pao surgery, and beyond /
  Jennifer Lesea-Ames, editor.

ISBN-13: 978-0-692-58520-7
ISBN-10: 0692585206

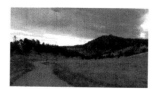

Warrior On Press
Lafayette, Colorado
www.warrioronpress.com

*This book is dedicated to those who are
living with chronic hip pain and to all PAO Warriors.*

Don't give up the fight.

Acknowledgments

The PAO Project and *Onward!* would not exist without the guidance and support of many, and for that, I hold heartfelt gratitude and love:

Karen Sudre, my sister, best friend, and PAO caretaker: Thank you for always being there with your unconditional love and support in this journey, whether it be caretaking, talking on the phone, or co-editing this book.

Erika Schreck, my dear friend, Reiki Master, and wing-woman for *The PAO Project*: I hold infinite gratitude for your unwavering support, insights, and talents with website design, book editing, and formatting. Without you, none of this would have been possible!

Jessica Dyke, soul sister and my first PAO buddy: Without finding your blog, my path would have been very different. Thank you for magical unicorn synchronicities and being there during my PAO preparation and recoveries. I have much gratitude for your willingness to contribute your editorial expertise.

Jenni Wong, dear one and the official PAO Cheerleader: Your positive words of encouragement and consistent support kept me going when I thought about giving up on this endeavor. Thank you for all that you do for all the PAO Warriors and for me.

Dr. Michael Bellino, my PAO surgeon at Stanford Hospital and Clinics: Thank you for your expertise, good bedside manner, and skill. I am forever grateful to you for giving me my life back.

The staff at Stanford Hospital and Clinics: Thank you for your professionalism, hard work, and care; you set the bar very high in patient care, and it does not go unnoticed. Thank you.

Karen Echery, my Physical Therapist, Lilly Miller, my P.T. Assistant, and the staff at North Boulder Physical Therapy: Thank you for your patience, your ability to push me to my limits but not beyond, and your ability to accurately assess my rehabilitation needs. I credit you for my normal gait and ability to get back to the physical activities I enjoy!

My family (especially my aunt Sue Yesilada and Grandma Vergie), friends, and the Periacetabular Osteotomy (PAO) support group on Facebook: Thank you for going out of your way to make my recovery easier. Words cannot adequately express my gratitude.

Evie, my beloved fur baby and heart chakra kitty of 14 years: I truly believe you helped heal me with your purring and unconditional love. I am eternally grateful.

Shawn, my partner in this crazy thing called life: Thank you for making me want to be a better person every day. I couldn't have done it without you. We are a team. I love you.

Table of Contents

Table of Contents *continued*

Chapter Four: Recovering From PAO Surgery

Chapter Five: Life After PAO Surgery

Chapter Six: Poems

Table of Contents continued

Chapter One
Living With Chronic Hip Pain

"If you are going through hell, keep going."
Winston Churchill

Editor's Note

Living with Chronic Hip Pain

According to the World Health Organization, "New statistics released by IASP [International Association on the Study of Pain] and EFIC [European Federation of the IASP Chapters] indicate that one in five people suffer from moderate to severe chronic pain, and that one in three are unable or less able to maintain an independent lifestyle due to their pain. Between one-half and two-thirds of people with chronic pain are less able or unable to exercise, enjoy normal sleep, perform household chores, attend social activities, drive a car, walk or have sexual relations. The effect of pain means that one in four reports that relationships with family and friends are strained or broken, according to the IASP/EFIC data."[1]

Those suffering from chronic hip pain are often misdiagnosed by health care professionals or attribute the pain to activity levels (i.e. running) or age. For 10 years, I attributed my chronic hip pain as part of being an athlete, taking on the mentality of "no pain, no gain." It wasn't until it progressed to a point to where I wasn't able to walk when I finally decided to seek medical attention.

In this first chapter, we begin the exploration of one of the common threads of hip dysplasia: chronic hip pain. Kris Amels' powerful narrative explores her lifelong experience with chronic hip pain, which was a stable factor in the trials and tribulations of her life, and the realization of what it would be like to be pain-free.

Daniella Whittaker, a talented ballerina, describes the progression of her chronic hip pain and the consequences of her pain while she received her formal ballet training in London. Additionally, she explains her determination to find an answer and a solution so that she may one day be pain-free.

Cammie Smith, a high school English teacher, explains that chronic pain has made her feel like a failure in many aspects of her life. Thanks to the lessons that her students taught her on her last day of work before her surgery, she realizes the opposite.

Natalie Davis bravely describes not only her experience with chronic hip pain but also failed surgeries and the aftermath of a personal tragedy. She is determined, like many, to find an answer to her source of pain and to live a pain-free life.

Colleen Lammers reflects on her journey of seeking answers and explains the toll that chronic pain took on her energy levels and personal life. She encourages others to be persistent with finding answers and advocates that early detection and treatment are keys for a long-term solution and a pain-free life.

Dawnelle Dutton, who was diagnosed with hip dysplasia in 2004, reflects on how the progression of her hip pain while being pregnant motivated her to seek a solution to fix her hip dysplasia.

Taylor Kulpa conveys how others were non-supportive of her careers goals because of her levels of pain. She refused to listen to them and pursued answers about her chronic hip pain so that she could pursue her education to be a respiratory therapist. She closes on the lessons learned through her journey.

Lastly, Sue Gombis' "I Am" explores how chronic hip pain and multiple surgeries have affected her as a person and her realization that chronic pain does not have to define her. She closes with standing in her place of personal power with her affirmations.

Kris Amels

It's All I've Ever Known

I grew up with pain. My hips have always hurt, always and all ways. I was born in 1968, and newborns weren't checked for hip dysplasia until 1970. My parents told me that I didn't even try to walk until I was about 18 months old. When I did, I waddled like a little brown-haired penguin in a pink vinyl dress—a small 1960s fashion plate with a drunken swagger.

Our neighbor from across the street, who was a nurse, watched me stagger around the front yard and said to my mom, "There's something wrong with that kid's hips. Take her to an orthopedist."

And so they did. After some X-rays in a gigantic sunny room that I recall smelling like vinegar and chemicals, in a huge office on Central Park West, I played with Dr. K.'s Dalmatian while he broke the news to my folks. Not only were both of my hips dislocated, but the sockets were also so shallow it would take years of treatment to fix them, so I could walk, and even then, I'd probably always have trouble with them.

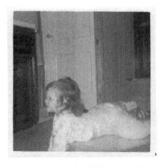

Treatment commenced. Surgery for tendon release. A year-and-a-half in traction in the hospital. I remember in my hospital crib, there was this horrible little musical pink kitten toy with a metal wind-up key on its back. Every time my parents visited, they would wind that toy up right before they left, and I would lie there, alone again and in pain, and listen to it as it played a tinny version of "What's New, Pussycat?" To this day, I still can't listen to that song, and even writing the title makes me feel a little nauseated.

Traction completed, I was sent home in a massive plaster body cast, covered from armpits to toes, with a cutout diaper window. The cast alone weighed 50 pounds. They changed the cast over and over as I grew. My father built a special chair so I could sit at the table. I remember my mom putting curlers and Dippity-Do in my hair, and sitting under her massive bullet hair dryer in that special cast chair while I had my lunch and waited for my straight hair to set in bouncy curls. My father also built a little sort of scooter—a crib mattress mounted on a board, with casters and a seatbelt, so I could lie on the board on my stomach and scoot around. A year of casts, maybe a little longer.

Another year of braces, huge leather and steel things, and I learned how to walk in them, wearing my fabulous 1970s red and blue polyester pants under the brace.

And then I was five. And there were no more casts, and no more braces. But my hips hurt.

And they hurt enough that I eventually learned not to complain about them anymore. I dreamed about not having pain.

And my parents tried to give me a normal childhood: gymnastics, ice-skating, horseback riding. I was good, too, a fast skater, and how I loved those big, strong, soft-eyed horses.

We went back to Dr. K. about once a year. When I was 10 or 11, he asked what I was up to, and I told him happily about the horses. I remember his big, bushy eyebrows slowly rising in shock when I described learning to skate backwards, and jumping my horse. After another discussion with my parents (though no Dalmatian for me to play with this time), there was no more ice-skating. No more gymnastics. No more horses.

But there was pain. That pain. The all-too-familiar bite of pain in my hip if I ran too far, or climbed a rope in gym, or rolled around on the metal floorboards in the back of the big blue Ford station wagon my mom drove.

So many things in my life changed then. My parents divorced. My mom became a violent, furious alcoholic. I became a ward of the state and went to reform school. My father married the woman he'd cheated on my mom with. I sued him for my child support after I came back from reform school, when I was homeless. I became an emancipated minor and rented my first apartment right after I turned 17. I became sexually active. And through all this upheaval... my hips. The constancy of pain in my hips.

I saw a new doctor about my hips, as Dr. K. had died a few years earlier. He suggested THR. I said no way; they weren't taking my bones out. That really disturbed me, the thought of losing my bones. Even though they hurt, and kept me from doing a lot of things, I'd be stuck with whatever they sold me prosthetics-wise. You can't go back once your bones are gone. Plus, that new hip was supposed to be replaced every 10 years. It was sold expecting to fail. I just couldn't get my head around that.

No, thanks. I'd deal with the pain. By now, it was my oldest friend, anyway.

Another apartment, this time in Brooklyn, a new boyfriend, a new job. Pain. All of a sudden, there were a lot of stairs in my day. To and from my apartment, the subway, and then I was on my feet all day at work. Pain.

And then, one day in 1996, an unwelcome surprise. I jumped out of bed, expecting to hit the shower and go to work, when instead I hit the floor. Literally. I jumped out of bed and landed square on my face. My hip had stopped working. I could bend my leg forwards but not back. It hung up in a straight line. I called in sick to work, and made an appointment for that day at Joint Diseases (the hospital I'd spent so much time in as a child). I hopped (literally) in a cab and met Dr. S. After a few X-rays, he said a bone spur had broken off and fallen into the joint. I was certainly a candidate for THR, but he knew of a new doc, one doing this PAO surgery—sort of sculpting a new socket from your existing bones. That sounded good to me, so he brought me over with my X-rays to see the new Dr. F.

Dr. F. took one look at my X-rays, one look at me, and said, "I can take away your pain." I burst into tears.

And so I signed on for that surgery. I was Dr. F.'s ninth Ganz osteotomy patient, in August of 1996. The surgery took six-and-a-half hours. And though I had plenty of post-operative pain (with my meds about half of what they should have been), the old pain was gone. He was right. He took away my pain that day.

And then a tall, sort of familiar-looking nurse met me in Recovery and asked me some questions about what day it was, and about my parents and my medical history (I thought she was asking to make sure I wasn't brain-damaged during the surgery). She turned out to be my nurse when I was a little kid in traction. Peaches was her name, and she remembered me. And I remembered her, too. She saw my name on the surgical list and ran down from the Peds floor (where she was now nurse manager) to Recovery to see if it really was me. She said, "Nurses always remember their babies."

I'd come full circle, from my pain's beginning to my pain's ending.

And now it's 2015. I never ended up going back for the Ganz on the right; before I could schedule the surgery, I had an accident in 1998 and fractured part of my spine, dislocated my SI joint, herniated a disk in my neck, tore some muscles in my back, and drove the screws from the Ganz into the sciatic nerve in my leg. They had to remove the screws, but the Ganz stayed strong.

Now I need THR on the right. My hip is in shambles, arthritic and abnormal, catching and locking, and the pain. Oh man, pain. I remember you.

But that Ganz hip... it's got some problems, but Dr. F. was right. He took away my pain. Forever. And I am forever grateful.

About Kris

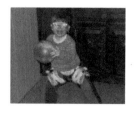

Kris is a fabulously frazzled frau, ex-reform-school kid, mom, and writer. At 46, she's still kind of surprised to have a four-year-old daughter. Both mom and daughter have hip dysplasia, but it's cool; they rock it. You can find her at www.facebook.com/WhyMommy or https://whymommyblog.wordpress.com when she has 10 minutes to herself. For a list of her books, please go to http://amazon.com/author/krisamels.

Daniella Whittaker

Hip Dysplasia, Dance, and Me

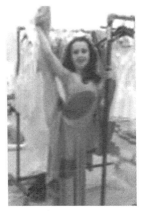

I started dancing at the very young age of two years old at the Fearons Middleton School of Dance. I can honestly say that right up until I was forced to stop, I loved every minute of it. I took part in lots of competitions and dance shows as a young child. When I was about eight years old, I auditioned and was accepted for the Royal Ballet Junior Associates. My mum took my sister and me to Leeds every Saturday for more than two years to take part in these ballet classes.

At the age of 11, I was accepted and awarded a full scholarship for one of England's best ballet schools: Elmhurst School for Dance (in association with the Birmingham Royal Ballet). I felt so lucky and grateful to be there, and I understood I was one of the few given the chance to receive such a high standard of classical training. I will always feel blessed to have been given the chance! Of course, this was a boarding school, so I had to leave home at a very young age, but it's only now that I see how big of a deal this was. At the time, it honestly didn't really bother me.

The days began at 8:10 a.m. and finished at 6:40 p.m. My place with the school was never guaranteed, and the end of each year brought an appraisal, which could lead to being asked to leave if I did not maintain the high standards required. In my second year at the school, I was chosen to dance with the Birmingham Royal Ballet Company, which was an experience of a lifetime. It gave me an insight into what I could be doing as a full-time job in years to come if I worked hard enough. The school offered me so many opportunities, including performing for royalty, meeting lots of inspiring people, and being a part of many performances.

I guess now I should talk about these hips of mine deciding to be a pain. Although the pain started before, I will start at the point when I had no choice other than to stop dancing. As I returned to Elmhurst for my fifth year, I had my first hip operation; unfortunately, I haven't done a ballet class since.

I was very determined to dance again at the time. Although I was unable to do what I was at the school for, I managed to stay there until halfway through my sixth year—a-year-and-a-half of watching my friends take part in classes and performances. It was the hardest thing, but I still had hope I could get back on my dancing feet. Although I couldn't dance for my audition to stay at the school for the sixth year, they still offered me a fully funded place. After everything, the fact that the school believed in me enough to give me the opportunity stay for another year fills me with pride. When I decided I had to leave, I could no longer walk a few feet without tears piercing my eyes. Even though I was devastated, I knew I had no other option at this point.

Having seen five hip specialists and having had several hip operations, injections, X-rays, and scans, and having to leave the ballet school, I still had no answers, and no one knew what was wrong. I never tell people when I'm in pain and choose to put on an "everything is fine" act, although the people very close to me know when I'm at my worst. Overall, I'm a very bubbly, happy, and extremely determined individual. However, four years after the first surgery, I won't deny that the pain was tiring, and the fact I couldn't go out to the local shops without excruciating pain was frustrating and didn't offer me a great quality of living.

It was in November 2012 when I had my first appointment with Dr. Bankes, and finally someone was listening to me! Finally, after all those years of pain, I was diagnosed with hip dysplasia, which is a deformity of the hips. Dr. Bankes was able to offer me surgery, a left periacetabular osteotomy or LPAO, meaning breaking the bone, repositioning it, and putting in metal screws. Don't get me wrong—I did plenty of research into the surgery, but with the position I was in, there was no choice but to go through with it.

In April 2013, it was surgery time, and I was feeling extremely nervous but also very excited for the chance to live my life like a normal 19-year-old. Having left home at the age of 11, I lost touch with the majority of my Yorkshire friends, and then having to leave Elmhurst, unable to travel, I also lost touch with many of those friends.

I do, however, have a small group of amazing friends and an even more amazing family, so I'm grateful to have their support.

The first month after the operation, I couldn't dress and bathe or really do very much without help. I really don't know what I would've done without that amazing support group around me. I did make improvements every day, and with the help of physiotherapy and a massive amount of determination, by August I was able to go out and volunteer for a charity, and I even started doing bits of dance again.

It was then at the beginning of October, while going up the stairs, the sudden pain made me fall and has only got worse since. Alongside this, pain just as excruciating started in my other hip. Although it is really frustrating to be back in the position of not being able to do much and experiencing very sleepless nights, what I have now that I didn't before the surgery is trust in my surgeon that he won't stop until things are sorted. I'm waiting now to have an arthroscopy (key hole surgery), which Dr. Bankes is confident will solve the problem, and then the journey to sort out my other hip will commence.

It's exactly a year on the 15th of April 2014 since my LPAO (left periacetabular osteotomy), and I thought it was a good time to try and explain to people, the best I can, my journey. There are so many ups and downs to put into words, but I hope my story so far will be interesting. If I can help even one person, then it's more than worth it.

About Daniella

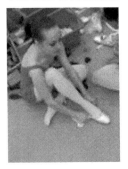

Daniella Whittaker, age 22, is from a small place in England, UK. She has a big, close family and an amazing boyfriend who have been with her through the many operations and ups and downs over the years. She writes about her hip story in the hope of helping someone else on the crazy journey that constant pain brings.

Cammie Smith

Elle est forte

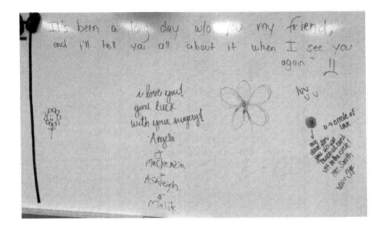

People who don't work in the field of education often make statements to me like "Man, I don't know how you do it. You must be a saint! There's no way I could work with teenagers all day," or "Teaching is a thankless job... the kids don't care and the parents blame you for their children's shortfalls," or "Sorry, that pitiful paycheck isn't worth the stress to me!" Or, even better, there are others who say, "Wow! You're lucky. You only work eight months out of the year and get off at 3:00 every day!" Most of the time, I just shake my head and bite my tongue to avoid conflict.

Is there some truth to those comments? Sure. There are days that are tough, really tough. There are days when I just want to come home, sit down, and cry. But then, there are days like today. When "my kids," as I like to call them, make me realize that there is no other job in the world for me other than to be a teacher... because being a teacher is my calling. Today, on my last day of work before my surgery, they showed up and surprised me with all of my favorite things: Oreo milkshakes, coffee, Chick-fil-a, Reese's cups, strawberry cake, Krispy Kreme donuts, cookies, and more (the sugar high was insane!). All of those sweet gestures were so kind, but the letters, the cards, the notes on the board, the hugs, and the encouragement—those are the things I will cherish as I begin this journey.

See, here's the thing. If I'm being honest, brutally honest, I've felt like a total and complete failure for the better part of two-and-a-half years. I'm in pain—bad pain—all... the... time. And that pain, no matter how hard I fight it, completely controls my life. I feel like a failure as a wife because I can't take care of my home and share responsibilities with my husband. I can't clean, I can't bathe our children, and I can't walk up and down the stairs to get pull-ups or jammies. I try to do my part by doing simple things like going to the grocery store, and I pay the price by being laid up on my back and icing my hip for the rest of the night. I feel like a failure as a person because I'm not fun to be around. I'm grumpy and snippy and tired after a full day of work. I feel like a failure as a mother because my pain makes me less patient, less understanding with my two-year-old and six-year-old, who are amazing children who often just do two-year-old and six-year-old things. I lose my patience and yell, and then hate myself for yelling, and I worry that I'm failing them as their mother. I feel like a failure as a teacher because I try so hard to do the best I can, all the while knowing that I need to be walking around answering questions, or helping students who are writing, but I can't... I just can't. It hurts too much. I've prayed every night for months that God will just help me move past the pain and be the wife/mother/teacher that I was before all of this started.

And today, on my last day of teaching, my students, my seventeen- and eighteen-year-old kids who are supposed to be learning from me, gave me a most precious, powerful lesson. I had some startling revelations while reading their letters and cards. A couple of weeks ago at church, our pastor showed us a commercial from the Dove company that was all about how we are so often our own worst critics, and how we see ourselves is so different, often so much more negative, than what others see in us. This was the lesson I learned from my students today. They said the following:

"You changed my life."

"You are an excellent teacher, role model, wife, and mother."

"You showed me passion for English and let me have a voice."

"You are such a strong person because you had so many things in your past that could have steered you wrong in life, but you chose the right track."

"You are a light to so many people in so many ways."

The icing on the cake was a painting one of my sweet students made for me. It says, "Elle est forte," which means, "She is strong" in French. On the back of the painting is Proverbs 31 (The Wife of Noble Character), and the note attached says, "Thank you for showing Christ's love to each of us through your teaching."

I have struggled so mightily these past couple of years with pain, fear, doubt, and

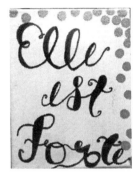

feelings of failure. These kids, *my* kids, showed me today who I truly am, in their eyes, and that has given me so much joy and peace. They have reminded me that I need to focus on the positive, the strength and passion I have inside me, and that if I do that, my light will shine brightly no matter how dark the road ahead may seem.

Five days and counting until my journey begins….

About Cammie

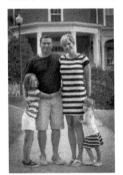

Cammie Smith is a 36-year-old wife, mother, and high school teacher who strives daily to keep God first in all that she says and does. She loves reading, shopping, and Reese's peanut butter anything. She played softball and danced for the majority of her early years up through high school, and she never had problems with her hips until recently. Cammie's dysplasia was not diagnosed until she was 34, after breaking her foot and walking in a cast for five-and-a-half months while she was pregnant. She had a right PAO on April 22, 2015, at Duke University Regional Hospital with Dr. Steven Olson. As she continues along the road of PAO recovery, her goal is simple: to persevere and overcome during this challenging stage of her life in the hopes of one day being pain-free.

Natalie Davis

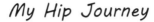

My Hip Journey

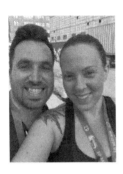

As a former ballerina and an active adult, hip pain was one of the most difficult things I have faced in my 30 years. I began my journey soon after graduating college. I wanted to grab life by the horns and use my newfound free time to get back into dancing shape. This came to a complete halt one day at work when I could no longer sit without constant pain. My coworkers, who were all clinicians, urged me to see a physician immediately. I did and was referred to an orthopedic surgeon who then diagnosed me with femoro-acetabular impingement. This is the diagnosis I would chase for the next four years.

The first surgeon took a significant amount of bone off of my femoral head, leaving it jagged. He stated a couple times that my femoral head seemed "too big" to fit into the acetabulum. After returning to the first surgeon, still in pain, I learned he wanted to take more bone. Before undergoing surgery again, I wanted a second opinion. I went to a second scope surgeon who said too much bone was removed in the first place and that he would only do soft tissue work which could help significantly.

Neither of these solutions helped for long. Both scopes had left my right hip severely destabilized and my surgeons scratching their heads. The second scope doctor simply refused to schedule another follow-up despite persistent pain and weakness. He sent me to three rounds of therapy, two of which were discontinued due to pain.

In the middle of all of this, I went through a deeply personal tragedy. My relationship with my partner ended after 11 years. I was devastated. I stopped eating. I barely functioned outside of normal tasks at work. I was a hot mess. After a couple months, I began to pull myself out and throw all of the leftover emotions into running. I didn't care if it hurt because emotions always hurt worse, and I couldn't hide them as well as physical pain. I was fabulously skinny and covering all of my feelings in sweat.

I maintained this until I accidentally fell in love again. I needed to deal with all the emotional stuff in order to fully move on. Getting rid of this baggage made the chronic pain scream out of neglect. Things went downhill physically for a while. I alternated between religiously stretching, ignoring the pain, and taking pain pills.

I went to my general practitioner. Just like the other doctors, she empathized with my situation, but she did something else: she tried. She wanted to help me. First, she set me up on Lyrica. This was so wrong for me. It made me feel fuzzy constantly, and the pain intensified. After the Lyrica failure, we tried a PM&R—this appointment was met with more doctor sympathy but a scratch of the head and another PT order. Clearly this was not the answer.

I somehow convinced my old surgeon to do an injection for relief. I needed to be normal even if it meant intra-articular injections. The injection gave me three months of much needed relief. I began training for a 5K. My new partner and I were flourishing together, and he was helping me pound the pavement. I ran a 5K on a hip that would partially dislocate from sitting down the wrong way. It hurt overwhelmingly, and that 5K was the last time I ran. My muscles never really recovered, and I spent the next six months in awful, nagging, constant pain.

I eventually gave up. This was my life now: wake up in pain, work through the day in pain, come home crying and exhausted, and lie on the couch the rest of the night. The routine was a stark contrast to my former life and, quite frankly, depressing.

My partner eventually got sick of seeing me in this cycle and insisted I see another surgeon. He found the number-one orthopedic hospital in our state, and I requested an appointment that night. I tried to be hopeful, but I had been so let down by the last three years I could barely squeak out an ounce of positivity.

My appointment day came, and I went armed with medical records and my armor on. I was prepared for the worst: that unmistakable glance at the X-ray and then a shrug of the shoulders with no help to offer. The doctor came in with nothing but a pad of paper. He barely listened to me, interrupting me as I answered the last question he asked. I was just about to give up on him and curl into the fetal position when he summoned me to go look at my X-rays with him. He pointed to my left hip and asked if anyone had ever talked to me about my dysplastic left hip. I was floored. I had been doing a small amount of research into the various Facebook groups for hip issues and knew a little bit about dysplasia—mainly the fact that I was very thankful I didn't have it. I tried swaying him to talk about my right hip, which was the one in agony, but he only talked about the left and explained that a more qualified surgeon in hip dysplasia can maybe see something on the right.

The main thing I took away from this appointment was a referral to the best surgeon in the tri-state area who could possibly help me. I made an appointment with him as I left the other office. I got an appointment but had an agonizing three months to wait. These months were very dark.

On the day of my appointment with the dysplasia expert (Dr. Z), I find myself not nearly as nervous as I thought I would have been. I am prepared for that big disappointment. During the examination, Dr. Z does all the normal range of motion tests, watches me walk and asks me when things hurt. Doc, breathing hurts at this point, but I do my best to concentrate on where the pain is originating. From the X-rays he has taken and my physical test, he has a theory: my acetabulum is over-anteverted. This means that my femoral head does not have enough coverage on the front of the joint, rendering it unstable. Then it's like a scene from a movie where all the pieces fall into place at once, and I am so happy there is a name and reason for all of this pain. While this is slightly different than dysplasia, it does take the same surgery to fix it: a periacetabular osteotomy or PAO. While there is a fix for this abnormality, it's invasive, and because of my previous surgery, he cannot guarantee this will put me back in a normal lifestyle, but he does think it can help.

I wait four more months for surgery. What's four more months when you've lived like this for four years? Well, apparently it is a nightmare. Waiting for this surgery is agonizing and stressful with unrelenting pain. Stretching no longer helps. I grow more tolerant of pain medications and have to increase the doses.

When surgery day comes, I am oddly calm, a welcome change from the last year or so. Since my time isn't until well into the evening, I have time to sit and think. I've been through surgery multiple times.

It's hard, but it is temporary. This day is the end of a chapter in my life. When I woke up, I began the next chapter: recovery.

The first two weeks I spent either sleeping, trying to sleep, throwing up, trying to poop, and just being plain miserable. One thing that did actually help was an agreement that my partner and I made before surgery. I had one goal at the beginning of the day and then one positive outcome from the day when he got home from work. In my darkest times after surgery, the positivity helped immensely.

After four weeks, the improvements every day made me feel more and more human. I could get around a little, groom myself, prepare a meal and accomplish some daily tasks. I was also weaning down on my pain meds. By six weeks, I was down to less than I was taking before surgery. This was a huge milestone.

I sit (yes sit!) here now 12 weeks post-op, and while I am totally exhausted, I am so hopeful. I have not felt that way in more than four years, and I have Dr. Z to thank for that—and also a set of very supportive parents, my partner, and a group of girls on the Internet who were always there when I was freaking out.

I will soon head out to PT for the day as I do three times a week until the end of the month. This past week, my perspective has changed, and so has my body. I no longer struggle to stand, my limp has almost disappeared, and I don't struggle through the entire day. Now, I haven't gotten to the point where I am no longer thinking about my hip—the achiness in all muscles and screw pain are a cool reminder—but I can see that day happening. Tears begin to well in my eyes when I think about the first day I am able to step onto the street in my running gear, headphones on, ready to battle the concrete. I know this will happen. I have to know this will happen.

About Natalie

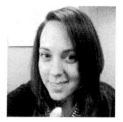 Natalie is a 30-year-old IT analyst and grew up as a ballerina. She lives with her partner, corgi, and two black kitties. She longs for the outdoors and an exciting, active lifestyle.

Colleen Lammers

My PAO Voyage

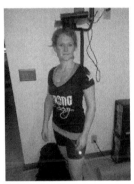

There are some events in life that change you. No matter how you may pick up the pieces, you will never be who you once were. Your outlook on life permanently changes. Looking back, what I thought were some of the hardest moments in my life, I now realize were a mere blip on the "toughen up radar." I hope to look back one day on my "overcoming dysplasia" journey and also view this as a tiny blip.

Prior to April 2012, I did not have any symptoms of hip dysplasia other than my ability to make a popping sound near my groin as you would cracking your back or neck. I didn't suffer from lower back, gluteus, leg, or knee pain. I have always led an active lifestyle; I'm a former rock climber, diver, runner, weight lifter, swimmer, and cross-fitter. I thought I would be one of the few that would grow into old age without a hitch. Actually, I was pretty confident of it. Looking back, I suppose we all think we are invincible.

When the symptoms started, they hit fast, and I quickly went downhill. There was no gradual decline; it was an avalanche. The takedown started April 2012 when I was 35. During workouts, I noticed knee pain. For a few months, I thought nothing of it and made sure to closely watch my form. Since the pain persisted, I requested that my Primary Care Manager (PCM) put in a physical therapy consult for me. The physical therapist diagnosed me with a tight IT band. Over the course of six months, my treatment consisted of dry needle therapy and corresponding workouts to strengthen the weak areas of my leg. The PT noted mild disuse atrophy of the left leg but assured me that once the tightness/trigger points were resolved, my muscle strength would come back. Sadly, it did not.

The atrophy worsened, leading to a left hip labral tear. Unfortunately, the doctors misdiagnosed the tear as a groin strain, and for the next nine months, I filtered through four different specialists while continuing with PT as the atrophy increased. The first hip orthopedic surgeon missed the dysplasia on my X-rays. Instead, he ruled that my hip structure looked solid and was not the cause of my pain. I was then sent to a rheumatologist and neurologist to rule out a potential diagnosis of myositis, which is a muscle disease. Both the rheumatologist and neurologist cleared me via advanced blood work and a muscle biopsy.

Meanwhile, as each specialist dismissed me, I still had pain, weakness, atrophy, and instability. Random movements would flare up the pain even further in my inner groin area and hip flexor area. The symptoms improved on some days, but most days were painful. As I progressed down the chain of specialists, different drugs were prescribed to help manage the pain. Dry needle was, and still is, my form of pain management. I did not want to be on narcotics with small children and a full-time job. I needed mental acuity to get through the day. Finally, I settled on a stronger version of Motrin called Lodine and Tramadol, paired with additional supplements suggested by a naturopath to help reduce inflammation. I also relied on massage, chiropractic care, and acupuncture to help manage the pain.

The roller coaster of emotions that accompanied me through this part of my journey was a struggle. Working full time, mid-career, trying to make up hours before and after work while managing pain, all while trying to be a mom and wife, exhausted me. Just getting through the workday was a chore for me. Most days, I was in tears by the time I got home, feeling frustrated with no answers, in pain, and trying to keep my life moving along. I wasn't the mom or wife I wanted to be. I missed so many sporting events with my kids, due to appointments and physical therapy or just the inability to go. The gravity of my situation really weighed heavily on my heart. How can a person in near-excellent health go from being on the go and active one day to suddenly in chronic pain and with limited movement and atrophy? It just didn't make sense... I wasn't satisfied with any of the answers the previous doctors provided, but I understood that they were trying their best to diagnose me within their area. I wanted a doctor that would assess the whole situation, not just the autoimmune, nerve, or bone. I may not have a degree in the medical field, but my background in IT kept me moving. I knew that there had to be a cause, and I wasn't giving up. I would not let this situation hinder my life. It might set me back on many levels, but I would keep digging.

That next step was to see a physiatrist who was finally able to diagnose me with a hip labral tear. From there, things moved along quickly. In addition to the labral tear, the second hip orthopedic surgeon I saw also diagnosed me with bilateral hip dysplasia. The doctor was honest when listing my options, informing me that if I chose the PAO route, I would need to seek a doctor who specializes in that procedure. After my initial consult with one of the top hip preservation specialists in August 2014, I had my LPAO on November 5, 2014, at Duke Regional Hospital. Eight months later, on July 22, 2015, I was once again being rolled into the OR for my RPAO.

From the time my symptoms started in 2012 to the moment that I met with the doctor that would ultimately perform my surgery, 28 months of my life had gone by living in chronic pain. Chronic pain at any age makes you feel cheated, but especially in midlife. By the age of 30, the majority of Americans are typically married, possibly with young children, while trying to climb the ladder in their professional career. We rely on our health in order to achieve all that needs to be done. The carefree life of your 20s is now gone, and in your 40s, life becomes more secure. You don't think in your 30s, "What if my health…?" That thought just doesn't enter your mind. That happens to older people, like 60 and older, but not in your 30s.

When trying to explain this surgery to others, the biggest question people asked me was, "Why subject yourself to such a surgery?" The answer is really simple. Having dysplastic hips is similar to driving your car across a poorly designed bridge. One day that bridge is just going to give out from the poor design and wear and tear. Dysplastic hips are essentially the same concept. One day, they are going to give out from repeated stress. One can try and train the muscles to force fire, but at some point, the joint itself is going to wear down, and osteoarthritis will set in.

Likewise, tired muscles become angry and create trigger points. These trigger points can cause a slew of problems: pain, atrophy, additional weakness, and so forth. This is why PAO surgery is recommended for people that have hip dysplasia. It sets the hip in the right position, structurally aligning our body, preventing any further damage to the joint, and thus relieves overworked muscles. Once the bone grafts back together, pain subsides by correct alignment and muscle firing.

Recovering from a PAO is a delicate situation because of all the ups and downs. However, dealing with a bilateral situation takes perseverance and acceptance, but most of all it takes patience and willpower. As I write this, three-and-a-half weeks post-RPAO, I can say with confidence that early diagnosis prior to the onset of symptoms is imperative. It doesn't take a medical journal article to articulate that early detection and subsequent surgery prior to the onset of muscle atrophy positively impacts post-op rehabilitation and reduces the chances of living in chronic pain. Although I am only a few weeks into my rehab, I can already see a different in my muscle control. I will continue to blog my journey as I progress through rehabilitation, hoping to live a pain-free life.

About Colleen

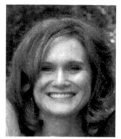

Collen is a wife, mother, and career woman. She is also fighting to overcome hip dysplasia and the subsequent pain that accompanies it. She is fighting to get her mobility back.

Dawnelle Dutton

My Hip Dysplasia Diagnosis

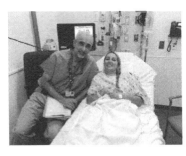

I was diagnosed with hip dysplasia in 2004. I was told that no options were available to fix it besides a hip replacement. I was also told no more running, jumping, or high-impact sports. At this point, I had just completed my first year teaching high school physical education. I finally saw an orthopedist who X-rayed my hips and was in dismay that I had been that long without diagnosis. At this point, I had had four big knee surgeries. Now, I knew these knee surgeries all stemmed from offset hips. Long story short, that day of diagnosis didn't really change much for me.

Sure, I started to think more about running and high-impact stuff, but being an athlete at heart, it didn't really make me stop. I got knocked down and picked myself back up many times on the court and field, so to me this was just a "speed bump," nothing more.

Then, at 30 I got pregnant, and this is where dysplasia hit me hard! I hardly made it through the last part of this pregnancy. I had regular doctor appointments for topical cortisone injections. After baby, things were better for a while, but then (and this was not planned), the second child came along. BAM—I was hit again. It was awful, and it was hard! I spent this entire pregnancy in physical therapy, trying to manage the pain. Then, after I had her, I knew I couldn't live this way anymore.

In 2011, I went to my local orthopedist and told her I was done and couldn't go on this way any longer. She gave me a list of two surgeons in California, and for no particular reason I chose Dr. Diab at UCSF (University of California, San Francisco). When I met with Dr. Diab, his main concern was that my two little girls could have dysplasia, so they were quickly screened. After following them for four years, both of my daughters were cleared, since no sign of dysplasia was found. Thank goodness—I definitely had that to be thankful for! I guess I hadn't even thought about my own children traveling this road.

My first PAO with Dr. Diab was November 2012 and the second November 2013. Both PAOs were eight hours or longer. Dr. Diab classified me in the top 10 of the worst dysplasia cases he had seen. My left recovery was rough as hell. My right hip was not as dysplastic as bad as my left hip. 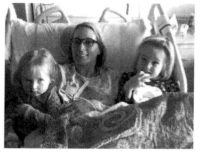 My right hip, however—which is my second PAO, hasn't healed like my first PAO. I have spent more hours/days in bed since 2012 than I could have ever imagined. My little girls were born unto a mom who they haven't seen any differently than one surgery after another. I haven't gotten too many days to sit down on my knees and actually play with them. I have pushed past a lot of pain to just enjoy them and be part of their active lives.

I've had two more surgeries since the first PAO on my right hip. This hip has been temperamental for whatever reason since the PAO. It's never fully been pain-free like the left hip. I've had one scope and one muscle reattachment since then, and I'm currently still recovering from the muscle reattachment. I cannot tell you what my future holds in terms of hips. I may have an actual hip replacement sooner rather than later, but I can tell you that it's led me down a path of rediscovery. I've rediscovered my purpose, I've become closer to God, I've learned to appreciate the blessings I do have, and I'm more willing to reach a hand out and pull someone else up.

My journey isn't over; it still continues. But it's one I'm willing to take because I know I have people by my side.

About Dawnelle

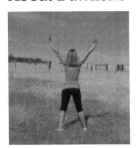

Currently 35 years old and diagnosed with dysplasia at the age of 24, Dawnelle was a high school three-sport athlete, college athlete, and fitness trainer/group fitness instructor. Currently, she is a high school/ elementary physical education teacher, high school varsity softball coach, and elementary volleyball coach. Dawnelle also runs her own fitness class and fitness boot camp business. Her most important current job is as a wife and mommy of very active five- and six-year-old girls.

Taylor Kulpa

This Is Not the End...It Is Just the Beginning

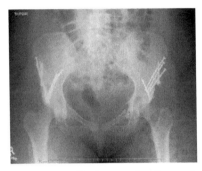

"You will need to drop out of college, as there is no way you can go into the health science field with your hip pain. I don't know what is wrong with you, so you just need to change your major and do things that don't cause you pain."

This is what I was told when I went into the many doctor offices to attempt to find out why I was in horrible daily hip pain. I could have accepted this as my fate and dealt with this pain for the rest of my life, but I knew that there had to be something else that could be done to help me. I set out to find that something! This is where my hip journey began.

After being told I would never be able to get into the health science field because I would not be able to stand for long periods of time, as is required in this career, I began seeking a doctor who could help me. Little did I know this was not going to be an easy task! I was eventually diagnosed with bilateral hip dysplasia and was told the only true treatment was a periacetabular osteotomy (PAO), which involved breaking the pelvis and realigning it over the head of the femur. Before actually going through this major surgery, I saw three specialists: one in Chicago, Illinois; one in Boston, Massachusetts; and one in Columbus, Ohio. I settled with the specialist in Columbus, Ohio: Dr. Thomas J. Ellis. What was so great about Dr. Ellis was that he was a surgeon who specialized in the hip and performed scopes, PAOs, and total hip replacements. He was the first doctor who put all the pieces together. At the first appointment, he said all the things the other eight doctors before him did, without me having to tell him my history.

Before I found Dr. Ellis, I actually had a right hip scope to repair my torn labrum and tighten the joint capsule. This was done in Pittsburgh, Pennsylvania, in May of 2013. I gave the scope a try before

I said yes to the needed PAO because I was willing to try anything before such a major surgery. The scope surgery only gave me about six weeks of relief, as dysplastic hips should never be just scoped, but I don't regret my decision to go through with the scope. Since this surgery failed, I had a RPAO in February 2014, a LPAO + left hip scope in November 2014, and then my final hip surgery in July 2015; this one was a bilateral screw removal and a right trochanteric bursectomy.

At the first appointment I had with Dr. Ellis, he noticed right away that I appeared to be double jointed. This led me to being diagnosed with Ehlers-Danlos syndrome (EDS), which is a connective tissue disorder that affects my whole body. Luckily right now it is only really affecting my knees, hips, and shoulders. Down the line, as I get older, more havoc will be caused by it, but for now I am lucky it isn't one of the severe cases. Having EDS made it even more necessary to get the PAOs done on both my hips.

I have learned several things over my hip journey these past two years, but the most important thing I have learned is to never take anything in life for granted because you honestly never know when your life will get flipped upside down. I could have very easily dropped out of school or changed my major, taking the advice of all the doctors prior to Ellis. However, I did not settle for that. I knew there was more to it than just hip dysplasia and that there would be a doctor out there who could help me. I was right. Dr. Ellis has literally given me my life back, and I will forever be grateful for him and his staff for all they have done for me!

About Taylor

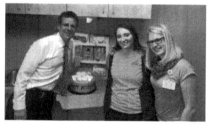

Taylor Kulpa is 21 years old and lives in Wheeling, West Virginia. She loves spending time with her two Yorkies and hanging out with family and friends. Taylor is in respiratory therapy school with a year left until graduation. She hopes to obtain her neonatal credential and work in a NICU in a busy city hospital soon after graduation. Since her surgeries, she takes nothing for granted, and tries to live life to the fullest everyday.

Sue Gombis

I Am...

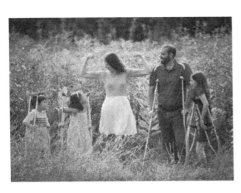

I was at dinner with some friends one night last week, still on crutches from my most recent hip surgery. I was in the bathroom when I overheard my friend, who was waiting for me in the hallway, talking with the manager of the restaurant about my hip drama. It was a bit surreal to hear his take on all this and the manager's honest reaction to what he was hearing. They were speaking without reservation since they had no idea I could hear their conversation on the other side of the door. To the average person, my story is unbelievable. I often hold back sharing too many details so I can spare people from having to conceal their shock. To me, it's just everyday life, and has been, for the past three years and the foreseeable future.

I have bad hips, really bad hips, if you were to ask my surgeon. Apparently I was born like that, but I remained blissfully unaware of that life-altering fact until I was 36 years old. After four MRI arthrograms, one CT scan, five cortisone injections, four arthroscopies (two on each hip), one open dislocation and rotational femoral osteotomy, one hardware removal, another arthroscopy and open dislocation (after an abandoned PAO), and more than 300 physical therapy sessions later, life will never be the same. It has taken me quite some time to be able to say that without bursting into tears; I've had to mourn the loss of the life I used to have. In the blink of an eye, gone were not only the obvious, like days of running as hard and as long as I needed to in order to clear my brain, but also the simple, like putting on a pair of socks and shoes without pain or struggle, driving a car without wincing, sitting with my legs crossed, and getting up from sitting on the floor.

I love to laugh, but spending years navigating this hip drama hardened me, and now I have forgotten. I became cynical; I found it difficult to trust people with my body, my pain, my thoughts, and my feelings. I felt broken and unfixable, so I reluctantly brought along pain as my sidekick in nearly everything I did. I felt completely lost. I thought my life had to be defined by hip surgeries, complications, and rehab. I was constantly a patient: at the doctor's office, in the hospital, at physical therapy for at least three times a week, every week, for years! When I closed my eyes, however, I still saw me. I finally realized that my circumstances don't have to define me; I get to choose what defines me. Carl Jung so eloquently said, "I am not what happened to me, I am what I choose to become." That realization brought me so much peace and acceptance with the fact that I was born with really bad hips.

My PT often jokes about how my next surgery will be hip replacements and how easy my rehab will be after all I've been through. While he is hopeful that I will not need them for another 15-20 years, he is quite certain that I will never be able to avoid them entirely. He asked me recently, "If someone could guarantee you that hip replacements would take away 100% of your pain, would you do it tomorrow?" I replied, "No." I have worked too hard the last three years to end up in that situation. I have set goals for myself, and I intend to achieve them one day. I plan to run again and to challenge my body to keep up with the things that my brain can dream of, like hiking Machu Picchu, running the Chicago Ragnar, and one day completing a half Ironman. I will not allow prosthetics in my hips to keep me from dreaming all that I can dream. Besides, as far as my surgeon is concerned, my last three surgeries have made my hips more functional, so I am allowing my brain to go wherever it pleases when I think about what life will look like when I finally reach my "one day." I still have to be careful not to get too far ahead of myself and concentrate more on the here and now.

I have lost a lot of muscle and coordination from the trauma to my joints from having so many surgeries in such a short period of time. My body has become a master of compensation, and my PT believes my body is completely unique in the way it decides to compensate. Typical exercises and rehab methods are often ineffective, sending him in search of new, creative ways to teach my brain how to use my muscles correctly. The process is frustrating and exhausting. While it is fun to dream of my "one day," my everyday still feels long and overwhelming. Recovery is a roller coaster: I can feel incredibly high one minute, after conquering a physical challenge, and in an instant, feel my lowest of lows when the pain becomes unbearable. I feel hopeful despite often feeling hopeless that my body will ever allow me to reach my "one day." Although I feel like giving up, I vow to keep fighting. In an attempt to help me cope with these daily challenges, people have said to me, "It could be worse." Yes, it could be, but my struggles are real, and I feel them with all my heart.

I decided that I just don't know how to give up when it comes to my hips, regardless of how impossible things may at first appear. I have tried—trust me—I have tried! I always knew I was stubborn and that I like to be in control. With that drive, that fight, that fire, I discovered that part of me because of my really bad hips. I found my laugh again. Although I'll never feel like the old me, I'm content with the me that I've grown into, and that is more than enough. I am strong, I am sympathetic, I am loyal, I am brave, I am a hip warrior. That is how I define myself.

About Sue Gombis

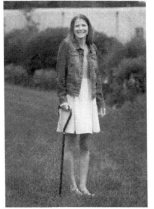

Sue is a mom of three little ones, a wife, an attorney, and a runner/athlete. While training for a half marathon in 2012, she injured her right hip and was diagnosed with FAI and a labral tear. Weeks later, she injured her left hip and was given the same diagnosis. Despite four unsuccessful arthroscopies in less than a year, her first surgeon abandoned her, leaving her to feel like her pain was not real. Sue was devastated. After a couple hours in tears, the fighter in her came out, and she found a hip preservation surgeon who validated her pain and diagnosed her with femoral and acetabular retroversion. Sue underwent an open dislocation and rotational femoral osteotomy on her left hip in April

2014. Because of the pain caused by the massive hardware, it was removed in October 2014. After a full year of rehab, she was ready for surgery on her right hip, an arthroscopy/PAO in May 2015. When the arthroscopy revealed cartilage damage, her surgeon abandoned the PAO and opted for an open dislocation instead. Sue is now in the thick of rehab, fighting to get her life back for her family and herself.

Chapter Two
Being Diagnosed with Hip Dysplasia

"Hip dysplasia, isn't that a dog's disease?"
a common response when told human hip dysplasia exists

Editor's Note

Being Diagnosed with Hip Dysplasia

According to the International Hip Dysplasia Institute (IHDI), "Approximately 1 out of every 20 full-term babies has some hip instability and 2-3 out of every 1,000 infants will require treatment." Additionally, "Adults with hip dysplasia is the most common cause of hip arthritis. A 2008 study from Norway showed that more than 90% of these young adult cases cannot be diagnosed in childhood by current methods of screening. This suggests that new methods for prevention or early detection need to be developed."[2]

When I was diagnosed with bilateral hip dysplasia at the age of 39, I was in complete shock. I, like many others, thought hip dysplasia only existed in canines! I always knew I never had a normal gait, but I wrote it off as a muscular imbalance until I received my diagnosis of hip dysplasia. For me, I was very lucky that my diagnosis was quick and easy, determined by a local orthopedic surgeon who was able to look at the big picture when looking at my pelvic X-ray. Unfortunately, many cases of hip dysplasia go unnoticed or are misdiagnosed, leaving people to unnecessarily live for years in pain. Correct diagnosis is the first step towards a treatment plan.

This chapter focuses on the varying journeys of women (and a child!) who receive the diagnosis of hip dysplasia. Laura Ricci courageously describes her pelvic floor pain, which led her not only to a focus in her physical therapy practice but also to the bottom line answer to her pain: hip dysplasia. Beth Hall eloquently describes her quest to get a proper diagnosis. In her story, she details the multiple misdiagnoses she received, which led her to her correct diagnosis of hip dysplasia, and the relief she felt when she had the correct answer. Nailini Hooper conveys her timeline for her to be diagnosed with hip dysplasia, realizing that it can take months of failed pain management treatment in order to finally reach a conclusion for her hip pain. Christen Thomas talks about the progression of pain that drove her to seek medical attention. Once diagnosed with hip dysplasia, she describes her treatment and path of her recovery. Lastly, Kris Amels reflects on her daughter's diagnosis of hip dysplasia and conveys her perspective as a mother. Her daughter, Is, also teaches her a lesson in perspective about living with hip dysplasia.

I encourage those who have chronic hip pain to listen to your body and seek at least two to three opinions with orthopedic surgeons who specialize in hip preservation. You are not alone; if you are on Facebook, there are support groups for (human) hip dysplasia and periacetabular osteotomy.

Laura Ricci

Pelvic Pain, Hip Dysplasia, and Hope

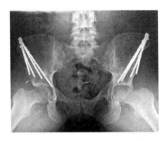

As a child, I remember my hips popping and clunking quite a bit, but it was not painful and didn't limit me, so I didn't think much of it. I just thought everyone's hips did that.

In college, I started running 5Ks and would notice that when I would go out for a run, both hips would ache for a full week afterwards, so I started gradually limiting my running.

A few years later, while in physical therapy school, I developed snapping hip and went to PT for six weeks. The physical therapist did everything he could think of, but it did not improve my hip pain with running and increased activity. I was told, "You just weren't built for running. Why not try cycling instead?" So, I took his advice and stopped running completely.

Two weeks after graduating with my doctorate from PT school, I married the love of my life, Mark. Once married, we realized I had a new issue: severe pelvic pain. I could not tolerate intercourse. At first, we thought it was because we were both virgins and inexperienced, but we quickly realized that this was not the case, and something was definitely wrong.

Here I was, 24 years old, newly married, and I was not able to consummate our marriage. I felt broken, like I wasn't a real woman. I felt alone and ashamed. I am so very blessed to say that my husband was amazing and supportive throughout this entire process. Together, we embarked on a very long pelvic pain journey.

I saw more than 12 doctors and tried many different treatments for the pelvic pain: pelvic floor physical therapy, Gabapentin, Lyrica, different creams, Lidocaine, hormones, Valium suppositories, and two surgeries (a partial and complete vestibulectomy), with little improvement in symptoms. Due to my own pelvic pain issues, I decided to specialize in pelvic floor physical therapy and took post-graduate courses to learn more in this area, hoping I could heal myself of the pelvic pain.

Eventually, my hip pain progressed until I had constant pain with walking, sitting, and standing. After seeing multiple doctors, I was finally diagnosed with adult hip dysplasia through a 3D CT scan of my lower extremities. It turns out I had a lack of anterior coverage caused by excessive acetabular anteversion, which is why my hip dysplasia was so challenging to diagnose and did not show up on a traditional AP X-ray. My PAO surgeon told me that 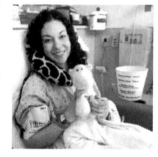 this type of adult hip dysplasia is extremely rare and only occurs in five to 10 percent of dysplasia cases. Typically, hip dysplasia shows up as a lack of lateral coverage, but mine was a lack of anterior coverage. In addition to the hip dysplasia, I also had bilateral labral tears and bilateral hip impingement. I had my left PAO on April 21, 2014, my right PAO on December 29, 2014, and bilateral hardware removal on June 17, 2015. Instead of repositioning for lack of lateral coverage, like a traditional PAO, my PAOs were repositioned in a different plane to correct the lack of anterior coverage. Looking back, I truly believe that pelvic pain was one of my first major symptoms of hip dysplasia.

I know, as a pelvic floor PT, that there is a HUGE correlation between hip pathologies and pelvic floor dysfunction, or tightness in the pelvic floor muscles. The pelvic floor muscles attach to the hips, sacrum, tailbone, and pelvis. Labral tears, impingement, and hip dysplasia can cause pelvic floor issues and pain with intercourse. My PAO surgeon told me that 50% of hip dysplasia patients will present with pelvic pain.

Sharing about my pelvic pain journey is not easy, but I feel like it is necessary to spread awareness in this area. If anyone is experiencing SI joint pain, low back pain, or any pelvic floor symptoms—urinary incontinence or leakage, fecal incontinence, difficulty emptying the bladder, pain with intercourse, pain with pelvic exams or tampon use, chronic constipation, low back pain, frequent UTIs or yeast infections, tailbone pain, vaginal pain, uterine prolapse, bladder prolapse, etc.—I would highly recommend seeing a skilled pelvic floor physical therapist, as NONE of this is "normal."

The pelvic floor muscles can become extremely tight before PAO surgery, due to overcompensation, trying to stabilize and make up for the lack of coverage and stability in the hips. Also, after a PAO, the trauma from the surgery and the adjustment of the bony alignment affects the attaching pelvic floor muscles and could send the pelvic floor into spasm.

Here are two directories to help find a pelvic floor physical therapist in your area:

- http://www.womenshealthapta.org/ptlocator
- http://hermanwallace.com/practitioner-directory

Please also know: this is a rare specialty, and many pelvic floor PTs have a long waitlist (around three to six months). It is my hope that we can get more PTs trained in this specialty because there is a huge need for this work.

It is my hope that by sharing my story, I can bring more awareness to pelvic pain issues and how hip dysplasia or other hip pathologies could be an underlying cause contributing to chronic pelvic pain.

Remember: trust your body and the information it provides you with, and never, ever give up!

About Laura

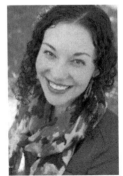

Dr. Laura Ricci is a licensed doctor of physical therapy specializing in Women's Health and Pelvic Floor Rehabilitation, as well as a certified Women's Health Nutrition Coach (WHNC) through the Integrative Women's Health Institute (IWHI). Through her own medical challenges, including cancer and major orthopedic surgery, she found a passion for nutrition. Since Laura had so much personal experience with surgery and recovery, she wrote and taught the Nutrition Pre- and Post-Abdominal and Pelvic Surgery course for the IWHI, due to her extensive experience in both areas.

Laura enjoys learning and expanding her knowledge in the areas of functional medicine and nutrition. She has completed a one-year certification in holistic health coaching and nutrition through the IWHI, and she is currently completing a two-year Nutritional Endocrinology Practitioner Training Program through the Institute of Nutritional Endocrinology.

Laura teaches nutrition classes and cooking classes, and provides private, one-on-one nutrition and health coaching virtually all over the globe: www.lauraricci.vpweb.com.

She strives to be a light in the darkness, offering hope for others with her personal story of love and healing. She lives with her husband in Amarillo, Texas, where she loves healthily cooking, going to Tai Chi class, and spending time in nature.

Beth Hall

Long and Winding: My Path to PAO

"Dinner's ready!" My mother-in-law's voice rang through the house at a family gathering. The smell of baking bread and roast beef drifted through the warm twilight, as I made my way to the table, one hand resting maternally on my abdomen, full with life.

Then, sudden, agonizing pain. I grabbed my hip and stumbled, shocked.

It was minutes before I could walk.

I didn't know then, but this was the beginning.

*   *   *   *   *

Her hair smelled as only a newborn's can, intoxicating and perfect. I nestled her sweet two-week-old body deep into my arms and drank in the view of her precious face.

We descended the stairs together: she slept peacefully, and I stepped gingerly as not to wake her. Slow steps on soft carpeted stairs.

My foot slipped, either in exhaustion or distraction, or both. We went down. In the economy of baby versus mother, baby wins. We were no different. My body braced tight, and I curved carefully around her, a mother cocoon.

My hips took the impact. Again, the searing pain came.

*   *   *   *   *

Three years passed. Now a young mother of four, my pain had spread. Terms like piriformis, sacroiliac, obturator nerve, and L4-L5 all became a part of my vernacular. The battle between pain and performance wore on. Days were lived in a grimace, in silent begging for relief. The rattle of acetaminophen—and eventually stronger prescriptions—became commonplace.

A mother smiles through pain. Her children need a good life. They never knew what those days at the park cost, those happy cries for "Swing me, Momma!" My body paid, but I smiled and kissed their milky skin.

When no one was looking, my body folded and the sobs came.

*   *   *   *   *

"We'll need an MRI of your brain. It's possible you have multiple sclerosis. Your right side is weaker than the left." (Neurosurgeon)

"It's 'mother syndrome.' You're just exhausted. It'll get better. I promise." (Sports medicine)

"It's most likely fibromyalgia." (Primary care physician)

"Have you considered cutting out gluten?" (Nutritionist)

"I can treat you three times a week for six weeks. It's $300 per session. No, I don't take insurance." (Prolotherapist)

"Sciatica." (ER doctor, on a visit when the pain was spasming)

"This won't hurt." (Needles. Tears.) (Cortisone injections)

"You're subluxated." (Chiropractor)

"Your aura needs to be realigned." (Acupuncturist)

"I'm going to try this technique called Bowen. I just lightly press my fingers every minute or so in various spots around your body. That'll be $135." (Body worker)

"Just use a wheelchair?" (Physiatrist)

*   *   *   *   *

"You have hip dysplasia."

His voice was calm and sure as he examined my X-rays, full of the diagnostic power I craved. My ears adjusted to his *sure*ness, like a tuning fork finding the perfect pitch.

Everyone else had been guessing, and I knew it. My body knew it.

My heart pounded. My breath seemed to catch in my throat.

I stared at the offending hip joints in the X-ray. Hip dysplasia, I thought. How simple. Could *this* really be the answer? How could he be the *only one* of so many to see this seemingly simple problem? The small exam room seemed to spin, unexplainably quickly yet in slow motion. His pen scratched against the X-ray, masterful angles and lines explaining how these uncovered, loose, unprotected hip joints had led to the size and scope of my pain.

There I sat, numb with gratefulness for the expertise of Dr. Mohammad Diab, UCSF pediatric surgeon and kind purveyor of the information for which I had longed, had begged for in the small night hours with tears salty and teeth pressed tight.

*   *   *   *   *

The surgery was scheduled: periacetabular osteotomy (PAO). My pelvis would be broken in several places and aligned properly, held together by titanium screws. The ensuing spaces would be filled in with donated bone.

It is one of the most aggressive orthopedic surgeries available. It is debilitating for weeks and even months post-operation and not uncommon for patients to still be treated and strengthening even up to two years post-surgery.

Yet to hip dysplasia sufferers, what price is there on a pain-free life? The PAO is a pathway to just that, paved by precious few surgeons in the U.S. and abroad who perform this highly specialized surgery.

I practically climbed on the surgery table and handed him the scalpels myself.

*   *   *   *   *

Almost a year has passed since my PAO. My story is not perfect, nor are my hips. Too much time passed without diagnosis for my hip joints and surrounding labrum to withstand the pressure of dysplasia, and irreversible arthritis set in.

But I am infinitely improved. Days go by without thought of hips and pain. I exercise daily and happily, enjoying the gym, gentle yoga, and long walks with my children.

My son is thrilled that I can get on a bike with him and pedal around with him.

Medication is no longer a part of my days. My heating pad, once a constant companion, has been relegated to a dusty corner of my closet.

Life is being *lived* again.

I am thankful.

About Beth

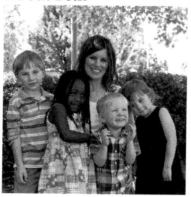

Beth and her family make their home tucked amongst the beautiful hills of northern California. She spends her days telling her four young children to practice their violins and floss their teeth, with a few other tasks thrown in for good measure (mostly involving sentences such as "Yes, you have to eat your salad" and "Please stop hitting your brother").

Her hip dysplasia has been both blessing and curse. It introduced her to a deeper level of connectedness with the suffering of fellow sentient beings, yet was also a source of sorrow for the inevitable losses that come with disability and pain.

Her great hope is for increased hip dysplasia awareness and prevention. She believes this book is a step in that direction, and for that she is grateful and honored to be a part.

Nalini Hooper

I'm Fine

I gratefully sink into bed. It's one a.m. and I'm exhausted. I worked for eight hours, mainly standing or walking. I hurt. My hips hurt, my knees hurt, everything from the waist down hurt. No wonder, I think to myself, "I'm the wrong side of 40 after all. It's normal to be sore after being on my feet all day." I think about taking some painkillers, but it's too much effort to hunt through the cupboard to see if I have any, so I go to sleep instead.

Six months later

I've changed jobs. I'm not on my feet so much and no longer work evenings. I'm on my way to work and reach for the ever-present Panadol (Tylenol) in the console of my car and pop two in my mouth before I start work. Two hours later, the pain is nagging and insistent, and I get a friend to give me two Brufen (Advil). An hour later, I pop another two Panadol to get through the next few hours. I collapse in a chair as soon as I walk through the door at home. Pain overwhelms me. "There must be something we can do!" my husband said for the one-thousandth time. "It's not normal to be in this much pain." I tell him it's arthritis and there's nothing that can be done.

February 1, 2015

I see my general practitioner (GP). I mention in passing my hips are sore. I tell her they're not really bothering me much, but she looks at them anyway. She diagnoses trochanteric bursitis. Hip pain is usually felt in the groin, and I have no groin pain so am reassured there's nothing wrong with my hips. She tells me I can have my trochanteric bursae injected, do physio, and my pain will be gone.

I get my ultrasound the next day, and they inject one side. I limp out after the injection. It's the first time I've limped, and it won't be the last. They also X-ray my hips while I'm at the radiology clinic. I'm instructed to put my feet in a neutral position for the X-ray. They're not happy with how I'm standing. As I look down, I notice my feet are pointed way out to both sides. That's how they've always been.

February 9, 2015

I'm at work. My GP calls me to tell me my X-rays show bilateral mild hip dysplasia. I've never heard of it. I tell her if I was born with it, it's obviously not causing any symptoms now since I've had it my whole life. She tells me I should see an orthopedic surgeon as "sometimes they do something about it." I make an appointment, but it's three months away, so I continue seeing the physio for my trochanteric bursitis.

The exercises don't seem to be helping much. I'm still taking painkillers to get me through a day at work. But I'm fine otherwise. I just need to start Pilates. Then, my pain will go away. I'm 45 after all; it's normal to have hip pain, isn't it?

April 22, 2015

I'm in the waiting room of my orthopedic surgeon. He looks at my X-rays and examines me and gives the nurse a knowing look when he sees my crazy range of external rotation and no internal rotation at all. I explain I can't put my foot up on the desk to do up my shoelace, as my hip will pop out. It doesn't hurt. It's always been like that.

He looks at my X-rays and tells me I have severe dysplasia on the right and moderate on the left. He measures some angles and explains them to me. It means nothing to me. He asks me what job I do, and I tell him that actually I've taken four weeks off work to get my hips properly settled down with physio and Pilates.

"You'll never get back to work without a hip replacement on both hips."

The statement hangs in the air. He shows me a model of a hip and explains the operation. Most of the rest of the consultation is a blur. I go home and act as if everything's okay, as I put my son to bed and host my cousin's birthday party.

April 23, 2015

My husband has gone to drop my cousin at the airport when I wake up. I feel hollow inside. Two hip replacements! I'm only 45! I take my son to school, and a friend sees I'm upset. We go for coffee, and I talk about needing two hip replacements and cry.

I go to another friend's house for more coffee. I cry again and talk about needing two hip replacements and how I'll manage.

While I'm there, another friend texts me and asks me how yesterday's appointment went. I text back, "Two hip replacements." Her response is immediate and in caps: "COME OVER FOR LUNCH." I talk about needing two hip replacements and how I'll manage and make plans for what I'll need help with. I'm not crying now. I've processed it. I go and see the secretary at work and tell her I'll be off for six months. I tell her how I'm going to manage everything. I'm fine. Everything is arranged.

April 29, 2015

I'm having a special MRI of the cartilage in my hips. They inject something into my arm and tell me to go for a walk for 10 minutes. I take the opportunity to run to my car, top up the meter, and run back. I have to sprint to make it in time, but I just manage it. My hips are aching a tiny bit after running so hard, but I know I'll be able to rest during the MRI.

May 20, 2015

I'm back for my follow-up appointment with my surgeon. He looks at my MRIs and is delighted. "I've got great news for you," he says. "You don't need two hip replacements. Usually by your age, your cartilage is so damaged that all we can do is replace the joint, but yours looks really healthy, so we can do a PAO on both sides."

The same feeling of shock descends on me. "Isn't that a bigger operation than a hip replacement?" I ask.

"Well, yes it is. But it's really good news…." He keeps on talking. I don't hear much. I go to the desk to schedule my first surgery with his secretary for the sixth of August.

I drive straight to a friend's house and repeat the crying and talking routine. They ask me why I should have such a big operation, when I could just have a replacement. I can't answer their questions.

July 1, 2015

I have everything planned for my PAO. I have a shower chair and raised toilet seat. I have 30 meals cooked and in the freezer for my husband to defrost. I have crutches. I have books and DVDs to keep me occupied. I have a recliner chair. I get a disabled parking permit. I don't use it. My pain is worse. I see my doctor and agree to start taking Panadol regularly. I've joined the PAO Facebook group and avidly read everyone's experience. I'm ready. I'm fine.

July 21, 2015

I see my GP. My pain is worse. I grudgingly agree to increase to one dose of Panadeine (Tylenol 2) a day plus three doses of Panadol. Since we have a shower chair anyway, I ask my husband to put it in the shower for me to use now instead of waiting until after my surgery. I can't stand for more than a few minutes without severe pain.

July 28, 2015

I see my doctor. My pain is worse. I'm taking two Panadeine four times a day and am waking up at night in pain. She asks me how I'm coping. I tell her I'm fine. My tears tell a different story. I only have another week to get through before the operation. She offers me morphine. I decline. I spend most of the day sitting in my recliner chair. Standing for more than one minute is excruciating.

August 3, 2015

My insurance company calls. They tell me they're considering this as a pre-existing condition, so surgery is delayed until March 2016. I see my GP. I ask for stronger painkillers. I'm constipated badly now. I start a pain diary.

My day consists of waking in pain. I take two Panadeine before getting out of bed. My hips are stiff and grumble, as I start walking around.

I take more Panadeine at 11 a.m., then Tramadol at two p.m. so I can manage the school pick up. More painkillers at five p.m. and again before bed.

I limp,
I ache,
I sit in a recliner chair most of the time,
I use ice packs and a TENS machine,

I can't wear high heels or do any exercise,
A 10-minute walk wears me out.
I'm 46.
Mums at school ask me how I'm doing.
I smile.
I'm fine.

Pain Med References
(Panadol= Paracetamol=Acetaminophen)
(Tramadol=Ultram=Tramol=Xydol)
(Brufen=Ibuprofen=Advil)
(Panadeine=Co Codamol=Tylenol 2)

About Nalini

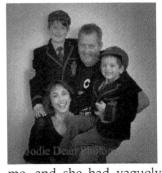

Nalini is 46 and lives in Australia with her five-year-old son and husband.

She has always been very active, dancing, skiing, biking, and doing gymnastics. Whilst she has had "funny" hips her whole life, she never imagined in her wildest dreams that there was anything wrong. She thought that having a perfect turnout at ballet was normal for me, and she had vaguely heard that dysplasia was diagnosed and fixed in babies by putting them in a "frog splint" for a few months.

She's looking forward to the day she can go out for a pain-free run and stop being the mummy whose hips are always hurting.

Christen Thomas

My PAO Journey: "You're Too Young for All of These Health Problems!"

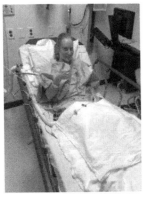

My PAO journey began when I was in my late 20s. I served in the U.S. Air Force for eight years and had been able to keep up with the demands of the physical activity. I had very little sports and fitness experience prior to enlistment, but I managed as well as could be expected. I was in good shape, not overweight, and made sure to exercise three times per week as required. I had been pregnant and vaginally birthed one child, and during and after the pregnancy, I noticed that my hips had started to pop almost every morning when I got out of bed and walked to the bathroom. I didn't really think much of it at the time and went about my life as a working wife and mother. Two more babies, discharge from the Air Force, working as a full-time realtor, and nearly 10 years later, my hip pain had progressed to the point of being unbearable.

In May 2014, after having my fourth child and struggling severely in my daily life to the point where I couldn't stand or walk for more than 30 minutes at a time, I scheduled an appointment at the Veteran's Affairs Hospital with my primary doctor. I asked for a referral to be seen in the orthopedic department for an evaluation. My appointment was scheduled for the middle of August (yes, three months later). In the time while I waited for my appointment, I continued to work and stay as active as I could with the restrictions I had from my daily pain in my hips. I had gotten so used to altering my activities that I found myself automatically declining invitations to go to places where I knew I was going to have to do a lot of walking or standing, including events at the kids' school, outings to the park or the zoo, and more. I realized I was missing out on being a part of my children's lives.

I was ready to find out what the heck was wrong with me and to find a solution no matter how hard it was going to be because I simply couldn't imagine going through the rest of my life with this diminished quality of life. I wanted to be able to go to the gym again, so I could lose the 45 pounds of baby weight I had just gained during my last pregnancy. I wanted to be able to work out with my husband at the gym and join him in fitness events, such as the Warrior Dash or Spartan races. I wanted to be able to go shopping with my daughters without having to sit down or leave after half an hour. I put all of my hopes on this appointment and was depending on the doctor to help me find answers.

My appointment was very enlightening. The doctor analyzed the X-rays and MRI scans and determined that I had bilateral hip dysplasia. While I was happy to finally have a diagnosis, I didn't really know what that meant. I was referred to the chief of orthopedic surgery at the VA, who then began working with me to find out where I would be able to find help to fix this problem, so I could get my life back. After hours of phone conversations and lots of research on his end, it was determined that I would have to go out of the state of Oklahoma to consult with a surgeon who would be able to help me with my hips. During these weeks of waiting and coordinating, I did my own research and found the PAO group on Facebook and started learning as much as I could about this diagnosis and what my options were. I also acquired my very own handicap parking permit (or as I affectionately call it, my "old person parking pass").

During my first appointment with my PAO surgeon in November, a 30-minute consult, it was determined that I was a good candidate for the PAO surgery. We scheduled my first of two major surgeries that I hoped would help get me out of pain and give me my life back. I was completely shocked at how shallow my hip sockets were and was filled with hope and a sense that everything was going to be okay. I knew it was going to be difficult, but I was ready to take the steps necessary to fix this health problem once and for all (at least for the next few decades). I got so much help and support from the PAO group online that I felt completely confident in my decision to press forward with this surgery.

My surgery was scheduled for June 2015. I passed through the spring season as easily as I could manage with my son's first birthday and making arrangements for my post-surgery care at home and was ready to go. Of course, as it seems to happen, life decided to throw me a curve ball and take out my primary caregiver with a broken knee two days before my surgery, so everything fell apart, and I had to regroup and change plans at the last minute, which is not something anyone wants to do. Despite all of the problems leading up to the surgery, the actual surgery went well and after a week, I was back home with my family to work on recovering.

My first week home was rough. But my husband was there to help take care of the four kids and me, which I was grateful for. Unfortunately, since neither of us was earning any money when we were home, he had to go back to work (as an over-the-road trucker) fourteen days after my surgery. Being left as the only adult in the house, I had to step up my game and get better so I could take care of the family and go back to work so we could minimize the financial losses. My 13-year-old daughter had to take on the responsibility of being the primary caregiver for the baby and did an astonishingly good job of caring for him and me in my third week after surgery.

I was up and driving 17 days post-op and back to work by 21 days. I smiled through the pain, and I spent a lot of time trying to explain the surgery to people who immediately thought of "hip replacement" when I said I had hip surgery. Those who wanted to hear about the difference listened to my dumbed-down, abbreviated version of what I went through, and those who didn't kept on thinking it was a simple replacement. But I was happy to be back at work. It was painful, but it felt good to be able to start bringing in money again. I tried to stick to my recovery plan as best I could and found myself pushing myself to 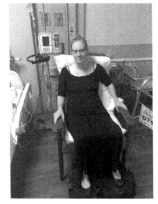 do as much as I could to keep the house running and the children fed.

Today, I am 10 weeks post-op. I am still in a lot of pain, but I manage. People at work have seen me progress from two crutches, to one crutch, to a cane, and occasionally with no walking aid at all. They offer praise and support in passing as we walk in the halls, and some still don't fully understand what I went through. It has been a difficult journey so far, and it seems like I haven't been able to catch a break. Nothing is easy. I know it is worth it in the end, so I keep pushing forward. Every day is still a struggle, but there is a light at the end of the tunnel.

I will have my other hip operated on in January 2016. I have no arrangements set yet for who is going to help take care of me, and I am dreading trying to ask for help again. There were a handful of people who stepped up and really helped out after I got home from the hospital, and I feel guilty for asking them to do it again six months later. It will be more difficult next time because it will be my driving leg that will be operated on, so I know I won't be able to get back behind the wheel nearly as quickly. I know I can't afford to be out of work for four to six weeks. What drives me forward is my aspirations and goals. I am not even 40, yet, and I have a lot left to do. I am tired of being inhibited by my body; I am ready to be well. I AM too young to have all of these health issues! And I am on the road to being rid of them once and for all.

About Christen

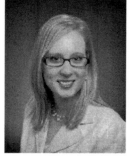

After battling with back and hip pain for more than 10 years, Christen had her first PAO surgery less than one year after her diagnosis in June 2015 and is scheduled to have her second in January 2016. She has a twin sister who has recently began experiencing similar symptoms as her own and is likely suffering from dysplasia as well. One of her three brothers also experiences hip, back and joint pain.

She currently lives in Norman, Oklahoma, with her husband Jessie and four children: Camille (fourteen), Gavin (eleven), June (seven), and Sterling (one). She proudly served in the US Air Force for 11 years and went on to become a successful realtor. After three years working as a realtor, she had to step back because the hip pain was so great she could not physically do the job. She worked as a Breastfeeding Peer

Counselor for the WIC program for just less than a year-and-a-half and returned to real estate after her first hip surgery in 2015. She graduated with her bachelor's degree in liberal studies from the University of Oklahoma in 2015.

Kris Amels

Perspective... and Popping Wheelies

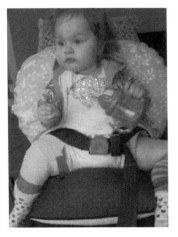

I have hip dysplasia. It wasn't caught until I was about a year-and-a-half old, and after years of treatment, it still affects my life in many ways. It became a part of my zeitgeist; it colors most of my personal history.

So when I got pregnant, I was already hyper-aware of all the risk factors for hip dysplasia. First baby, check. Family history, check. A girl, check. Big baby, check. Frank breech, check. My kid hit every risk factor.

When she was born, my daughter was folded up like a clam. Her feet had been wedged so hard behind her head; her right ear was folded in half. She also had torticollis, the angry stepchild of hip dysplasia.

The longest silence I've ever heard was when I waited for the doctors to resuscitate my baby. I lay there, split open and immobilized, while two surgeons tried to sew up my guts, two more doctors worked to unfold my baby and get her breathing. The nurses came over and held my head, trying to draw my attention away from what the docs were doing and saying. My spinal block had worn off long ago, and I was caught between floating on the 10 of morphine I'd just received, listening to the surgeon's breathy cursing over my abdomen, to the whispers of nurses and docs over in the corner with my baby. I focused on the corner.

Nothing.

No cries. No breath.

And then.

And then, finally, a cry. Small. Another: louder, bigger. And I knew she'd be okay, except for her hips.

The nurses wrapped her up, and held her damp face up to mine for a kiss, then whisked her away to the special needs nursery. That was her first day.

Her second day, my daughter, Isobel, after being seen by the local pediatric orthopedist, was diagnosed with bilateral hip dysplasia and was fitted with a Pavlik harness. Fortunately, he had one in the trunk of his car. Both hips were dislocated.

I got good at cuddling her, bathing her, feeding her and changing her around that ever-present harness. It cut into the soft baby folds of her neck. I applied diaper cream and wrapped thin, soft flannel strips around the shoulder straps.

When she fell asleep in her bassinet, I gently turned her head to the left, to relax those muscles in her neck and kick that torticollis's butt.

Two weeks later, we took her to see Dr. F., the surgeon who'd done my Ganz osteotomy back in 1996. He pulled off the Pavlik, checked Isobel's hip with ultrasound, and told us her left hip was in the socket; the Pavlik had worked, at least half way. The right hip would need more work.

I had to keep this in perspective. Hips can be fixed; it's mechanical. Her heart was okay, as well as her lungs. I could help her with her hips. I knew what I was dealing with; hip dysplasia was something I understood. I kept saying it to myself like a mantra: "Perspective."

I knew what she could be in for if we didn't stay on top of her treatment. Dr. F. wanted an arthrogram at three months, under sedation, to see what was going on with her right hip. She was so tiny. They did it at NYU instead of Joint Diseases, "in case something goes wrong" (which is totally not what any parent ever wants to hear).

Nothing went wrong.

Perspective, right?

When they wheeled that giant crib into recovery, I followed behind it like a magnet. The nurses asked my husband and me to wait out in the hall until they called us; I said okay and stayed where I was. They asked again, and I said okay again. But I couldn't move my feet to leave my baby. I stayed out of the way, but within sight of my daughter. Not soon enough, I got to hold her again.

Her right hip would take more work, but they would wait until she was six months old to try a closed reduction and spica cast. In the meantime, she was in a Von Rosen brace, which kind of looked like a yellow Gumby doll holding her from behind.

When she was six months old, we went back to the Hospital for Joint Diseases. We had to be there at six in the morning. Isobel (or Is, as we call her) was amazingly calm, looking around, smiling at people. The surgery took a few hours, so my husband and I chose to fret over cups of tea in the sunny cafeteria instead of the windowless basement waiting room. Soon our little buzzer from the operating service rang, and we ran back down to the basement to wait outside recovery for Is.

She came out of the operating room in a huge white cast. I got busy lining the edges with moleskin while she slept off the anesthesia.

They'd done a closed reduction, and she'd be in the spica for a few months. We stayed over in the hospital for one night. Is didn't seem to mind the cast. We spent a lot of time sitting around with her on our laps, reading and playing music.

She came out of the cast about two months later, and her hip still wasn't in the socket.

They waited until she was a year old, and tried an open reduction, where they cut the hip open and try to seat the femoral head in the acetabulum. It wouldn't go in. There was soft tissue in the socket, so they removed it, seated the hip, and casted her again. We stayed overnight again. She was in the cast for about two months, and they removed the cast the week before Christmas. She seemed happy about getting around and tried to stand up the day they took the cast off.

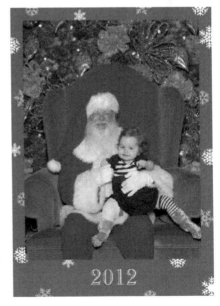

Isobel was getting really good with her fine motor skills, but her gross motor skills were lacking; she fell over a lot, and it was hard for her to stand up for any length of time. Those casts were taking a toll on her abdominal and back muscles.

On Christmas morning, she sat on the couch and opened her gifts. She seemed a little out-of-sorts, which was odd, because she was usually so happy.

When I tried to change her diaper, she screamed when I touched her leg. I knew something was terribly, terribly wrong. I called the hospital; we packed up Is and drove into the city. An X-ray showed her right hip was out of the socket. Again.

They think she dislocated it in her sleep. We spent Christmas Day in the hospital, and she had a closed reduction the next day plus two more months in the spica.

Her gait was still a little weird even though she was in physical therapy. At around 18 months, she went in for a femoral osteotomy, to turn the femoral head back, so it would seat better in the acetabulum. Two more months in a spica.

I was like a spica ninja by now: I had that spica care and diapering thing DOWN. I had a spica kit I brought to the hospital with me: scissors, Moleskin, duct tape. When the doc took the cast off, he looked at the cast, then back at me and said, "Man. That's the cleanest cast I've ever seen."

At around three years old, they took the femoral hardware out. She didn't have a cast after, but she was supposed to spend six weeks non-weight bearing. We got her a wheelchair and about 50 gallons of Legos. We popped wheelies in the chair and built Lego sculptures.

At around three-and-a-half years old, I noticed her gait was off again. She was throwing her right leg out in a circle when she ran with the other kids on the playground. Back to Dr. F.

Her hip was subluxed, so back to the operating room for another open reduction, four days in the hospital, and almost three months in spica casts. She came out of the last cast in May. Now it's August. She's had aqua therapy, which she loves, three times a week. Her gait is straight and strong, and her stamina is amazing. Yesterday she rode her Big Wheel for almost a mile. Through everything, she's been a smiling, happy kid: it's like she's a rock star at the hospital. Everyone knows her, and everyone stops to say hello.

I asked Is yesterday what she thought about having hip dysplasia and how it's affected her life so far. She thought about it for a few seconds and said, "It was really fun to pop wheelies in my wheelchair."

So there you have it. It really is all about perspective.

About Kris

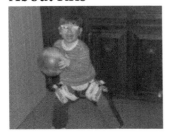

Kris is a fabulously frazzled frau, ex-reform-school kid, mom, and writer. At 46, she's still kinda surprised to have a four-year-old daughter. Both mom and daughter have hip dysplasia, but it's cool; they rock it. You can find her at www.facebook.com/WhyMommy or https://whymommyblog.wordpress.com when she has ten minutes to herself. For a list of her books, please go to http://amazon.com/author/krisamels.

Chapter Three
Preparing for PAO Surgery

"Hope strengthens, fear kills."
Karen Marie Moning

Editor's Note

Preparing for PAO Surgery

Periacetabular osteotomy (PAO) surgery has been regarded as one of the most invasive and complex elective orthopedic surgeries in existence, with a long rehabilitation period. It certainly is not for the faint of heart. Once the decision has been made to have this surgery, a lot of physical, mental, emotional, and financial preparations are necessary.

In this chapter, "Preparing for PAO Surgery," we begin with a narrative essay unlike the others: Gregory Lammers' is one from the perspective of the caretaker. He explains the importance of the caretaker's role, the lessons that he has learned from his wife's PAO recoveries, as well as some suggestions for future caretakers. My narrative essay reflects on the similarities between a warrior and one preparing for treatment. Originally a blog post that I published in January 2014 was the catalyst of the term "PAO Warrior," which is referenced throughout this anthology. Jessica Dyke's story explores the mental preparation for her second PAO surgery and reflects on her internal shifts after her first PAO surgery. Jill Campbell describes how the pieces fell into place for her PAO surgery, all while juggling the responsibilities of motherhood and working with her husband's military schedule. Annie Swanberg's story conveys the internal struggle with taking a leap of faith in order to have the surgeries that would give her her life back. The last "story" is my practical blog post and checklist for the items that I used at the hospital and for surgery recovery.

These stories give a snippet of what PAO preparation involves, and it's different for everyone. It is best to think of PAO preparation as a Venn diagram, with each aspect of preparation affecting the other:

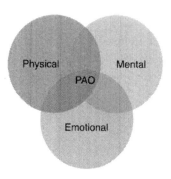

Preparation for PAO surgery is more than just obtaining the necessary equipment (e.g. shower chair) for surgery recovery. One must prepare the mind and manage the pain until surgery day.

Gregory Lammers

Hip Dysplasia Is Not an Individual Diagnosis

Hip dysplasia is not an individual diagnosis. This is a family diagnosis. Hip dysplasia is serious enough that the family life is going to change.

I am the husband to a wonderful woman who was living in pain. I marvel at her persistence to find out what was wrong.

We are in this together. Twelve years ago, I married the woman who makes me laugh, makes her own money, and loves roller coasters (the advice I give our three little boys on their future girlfriends/wives).

This is my side of the story as a spouse of a double recipient of a periacetabular osteotomy (PAO). I do not remember when she first started talking about the pain. I do remember when the pain really began. In December 2013, she started complaining about pain in the groin, and I, like the doctors, wrote it off as a pulled muscle. The doctors doubted her, and at times I doubted her too. I kept iterating to her that it takes time to heal. By spring, the pain did not get much better. I began to wonder if there wasn't more to her issues. Maybe time was not going to heal her. I noticed she had more doctor appointments. I noticed she began to see more specialists. I attended more appointments to provide support.

I distinctly remember when she finally had an answer. A brilliant orthopedic surgeon about 30 minutes from the house looked at her X-rays and watched her walk and said, "You have bilateral hip dysplasia." The drive home was quiet. I was happy for her that she finally had an answer. The next few months went quickly. I know the three-and-a-half-hour drive to Duke Regional Hospital very well. I joke with her that "I love spending all my vacation time in Durham, North Carolina," but I would not have it any other way.

I know the feeling, in my 30s, to sleep in a hospital chair while the woman I love is in so much pain. I know what it feels like having to dress a grown woman. I saw the difficulty she had doing the simple activities we normal folks take for granted. I lived through taking care of my significant other when she was not capable of taking care of herself. I truly felt at times I was taking care of a grown infant. I know what it feels like to be considered an afterthought.

Having dysplasia is not cheap. I have spent enough money to start my own massage business on anatomy books, foam rollers, massage balls, heating pads, ice packs, and one Bio Mat. I feel like I have put a chiropractic doctor's and dry needle specialist's children through a year of college. There are hotel rooms, gas mileage, and car maintenance. I would do it again without skipping a beat.

Through all of this, I am a stronger person. I have spent an enormous amount of time trying to remain positive and encouraging. There are days I do it better than others. As a spouse, I can only take in so much.

There are days I feel the family rests on my shoulders. Some days I cannot keep up, and that is okay. There is always tomorrow. I am either the little train that could: "I think I can, I think I can." Or, I am Dory: "Just keep swimming. Just keep swimming."

What have I learned through all this?

You cannot do this by yourself. You need a list of professionals to help you and your significant other through this. Be conservative with your healing, and err on the side of caution.

You need to have an open dialogue. You need to have a code word that can be used when you or your significant other can use to be heard. You need to be open with children. They are a lot smarter than we take them for.

Sometimes the only people you can count on are those in your household. Most people do not understand the complexity of the procedure or the healing process. Most people will isolate you. You will find out who your true friends are.

You must truly evaluate what is important to you. Work-life balance is tricky—even trickier if you need the work to pay for the procedure.

You must understand insurance and not just medical insurance but disability insurance as well.

All said and done, I want us to have a life together with her free of pain. I want us to cross off some of the items on our bucket list, but if we can't, that is OK because I married the woman that makes me laugh.

About Gregory Lammers

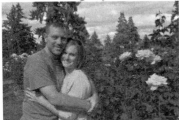

Gregory Lammers, husband to Colleen Lammers and father to three little boy clowns…

Jen Lesea-Ames

Warrior

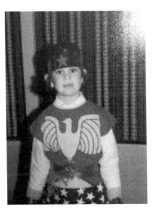

I have my routine in the mornings: I love to wake up around 5:30 a.m., pad to the kitchen in my soft slippers, feed the cat, make a pot of coffee, drink an Emergen-C, and hop on my email and Facebook. I was scrolling through my Facebook feed this morning and read a post from a friend of mine whose good friend, who appears to be around my age, was diagnosed with stage IV pancreatic cancer that metastasized to the liver. This struck a chord with me, as it is the same cancer that my dad was diagnosed with in 2004. Beyond the initial shock and sorrow, I thought about how my hip dysplasia and upcoming surgeries pale in comparison to her battle. Then my mind wandered….

And I thought, "No matter the nature of our health battles, be it cancer, hip dysplasia, or another disease, we are warriors."

To me, being a warrior is encompassing a certain mind frame and the determination to fight and push back at the disease. While we are prone to feelings of self-pity (we are human, after all), warriors allow the feelings to come, honor them, release them, and move on. Warriors prepare in every aspect of getting ready for battle, through scheduling doctor appointments, fighting with health insurance companies, asking questions, asking more questions, arranging a support group (rallying our troops), ordering necessary medical and/or health equipment, and handling logistics of all ends of the spectrum.

Warriors have a strong mind. We are determined to do anything and everything to improve our state of health. When it's time for surgery, warriors step into the hospital courageous and positive. After all, the warrior and her troops (in this case, the surgical team) are prepared. Warriors are determined to do anything and everything to get back their health, from physical therapy to follow-up treatments. A warrior's will is unwavering, and warriors dig deep within themselves to find strength.

When I find myself being upset about my condition, upcoming surgery, and rehabilitation, I remind myself that I am a warrior. It's empowering. That reminder enables me to keep pressing on to be strong, positive, and fearless.

About Jen

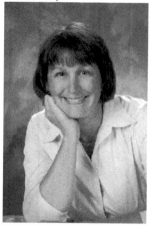

Jen lives her life with a passion to make a positive impact in this world. She is an exercise physiologist by training, a metalsmith jewelry artist, and a former triathlete. Diagnosed at the age of 39 with bilateral hip dysplasia, she had two PAOs in 2014 with Dr. Michael Bellino at Stanford Hospital and Clinics. She is currently enjoying a pain-free life, and it's her mission to help increase awareness of hip dysplasia and PAO surgery by sharing our journeys.

Jessica Dyke

In-Between PAO Surgeries

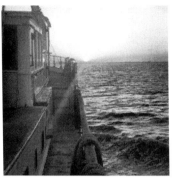

I rolled out of my bunk at five a.m. this morning, pulled on my boots, and dragged myself up to the deck. As I squatted down to loosen the starboard bowline, I contemplated my life and my body. I watched the 60-year-old engineer limp across the deck, and I thought to myself, "I feel you, buddy." I love boat work, but my hip does not.

The research vessel *Polaris*, originally a yacht built in 1927, is full of little staircases and ladders that connect multiple levels from the bunkrooms to the upper "poop" deck. It's quite charming, but I find that my hip has a hard time with so much climbing, stooping, and crawling. It's a reminder that while my hip is much improved from its pre-PAO condition, I still have limitations. I've been dabbling in some relatively high-impact activities, but I find that my body still prefers gentler activities like bike riding around town, swimming, and Pilates. When I do flare up, I typically feel much better after a day or two of rest. It's been one year since my left periacetabular osteotomy (PAO), and I find myself wondering if I'll ever be able get back to the way things were before my hip pain began. Are my days of hardcore snowboarding over? Do I just need to be patient and give my body more time?

As I type this, my operated hip throbs off and on in the pubic bone/hip crease region. I can't tell if it's trauma within the joint space or the area where the pubic bone was cut through. The muscle in the upper-outer part of my thigh has been stiff and sore every day since surgery, and I still have a partially numb area on my outer hip. Also, my TFL and gluteus medius are constantly tight and sore. I am by no means pain-free, and perhaps I may never be. My LPAO surgeon once told me that my pre-LPAO hip arthritis was at a level 2 (on a 0 to 4 scale), and I could expect to feel a big improvement with a PAO but that I would likely still feel some pain after a tough workout, such as a long day of snowboarding. I need to accept that and adjust my expectations accordingly. I also need to remember that my body experienced major trauma during the PAO procedure, and I suspect that it may take more than a year for my body to fully recover and find its new baseline. Despite the lingering surgery-related pain, I do think my left hip is up to the task of bearing the brunt of my weight while I recover from my upcoming right PAO. I've gotten most of my muscle back, and I feel strong. The pain in my right hip joint isn't too bad yet (level of arthritis unknown), so I'm hoping I will recover more quickly and with less pain the second time around. Plus, I think it will feel good to bring my body back into balance. My left hip joint center-edge angle was shifted from about 11 degrees to 35 degrees (within the normal range), while my dysplastic right hip still sits at about 11 degrees. I'm cockeyed! I'm very interested to see how different my healing experience will be the second time around with a new surgeon and slightly different protocols.

I'm writing while sitting in the fantail of the *Polaris*. Because of my hip issues, I haven't been out on the water much over the past couple of years. I have greatly missed it. I appreciate every moment I spend on the water today—the low roar of the diesel engines, the calming effect of being surrounded by water, the way it shifts 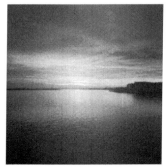 and resets my energy, the five a.m. wake-up call, watching the full moon set from the wheelhouse, standing aft in the steady wind, hosing mud off the decks, the colors cast upon the landscape as the sun emerges over the horizon, the creaking lines, the winch motor oil oozing into a puddle on the deck, pissing into a waxy envelope and "flushing" it down the Incinolet, the gentle rocking of the ship in the waves, the Golden Gate Bridge with the open ocean just beyond, the San Francisco cityscape, peeping through old-school portholes, staring up at the steel beams comprising the underbelly of the Bay Bridge. It has been the best part of my nine-year stint as a hydrologist at the USGS, and I'm incredibly grateful for every single cruise I have attended. I smile as I silently broadcast my private farewell, and it is bittersweet.

It's not officially my last cruise, but I know in my gut that I won't be back. My right PAO is two weeks from today, and I hope to have moved on to a new job before I am physically ready for boat work again. I say this knowing full well how dangerous it is to put my life on a timeline. Expectations and timelines have been the recipe for so much disappointment over the past couple of years. Going into my first PAO a year ago, I assumed I'd be a fast healer, that I'd have PAO number two within six months, that within a year I'd have both PAOs and recoveries behind me. I had always been so robust and healthy, and I prided myself in my physical prowess. So why did it take me nine long months to heal my bones? It's been difficult being patient and letting my body set the pace. The biggest lesson I've learned in the year since my LPAO is that sometimes you need to surrender to life as it presents itself and just warrior through.

In the vise grip of this hip saga for over two-and-a-half years now, I have often felt battle weary, deflated, my spirit fully contracted. But in the past three months since my multi-fractured pelvis was declared "healed," I have felt my spirit coming alive again, gaining vitality, kind of like in that movie *Pleasantville* when the black-and-white world starts spontaneously erupting in vibrant colors. I have thrown myself into living life with the sort of carefree, fun-loving humor and sense of spontaneous adventure that was lost to me for so long. This reprieve has been healing to my spirit and my sanity, but I still have so much pent-up wildness within me. I want to hike on rugged terrain in the dark of night, strip naked and dive into a moonlit lake. I want to leap and dance, bare feet on damp earth, wind whipping through my mane. I want to rip off clothing and kiss warm, salty skin. I want charge down steep, rocky trails on my mountain bike. I yearn to be back on my snowboard, shredding through a celestial sea of perfect powder, caressing every curve of the mountain. Deep in the trees, I find the clearest path into my heart.

I know that an essential, fierce piece of me is aching for revival, but I need to contain it, hide it away into a lockbox deep in a dusty corner of my soul. Right now, I must warrior up for the battles ahead.

My bone-shifting, soul-shifting journey over the past year has transformed me. I had my pelvis sawed apart, shifted, and screwed back together again. That is just the physical part of this process; my life, my dreams, and my identity have all been fractured as well. I'm not the same as I used to be—structurally and spiritually—and I am still on a journey through the innermost dimensions of my mind waves, undergoing internal metamorphosis. Who am I? Perhaps more importantly, who do I want to become? I've learned that there is a great freedom in losing the persona and the life that once defined me. I'm on the verge of a major paradigm shift, and I have the freedom to redefine my existence. I see this time of my life as a profound turning point. As I approach my second periacetabular osteotomy, I'm busy again building my cocoon, my fertile chrysalis, preparing for the next round of personal growth. I welcome the challenge. The pain will be my healing. I am ready to bring my body and my life back into balance.

About Jessica

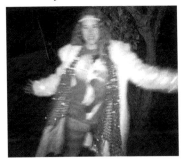

The Juicer is a warrior. She is a seeker of adventure, depth, and truth. She stares intently into the abyss, dreaming of intriguing possibilities. She will boldly step into the flames and let the fire burn away the debris. She is tectonically shifting into a life beyond her wyldest fantasies.

Her hip saga began on August 21, 2011, when she tore her labrum while backpacking on the northern California coast. Since then, she has had two PAOs by two different surgeons in 2013 and 2014, one screw-removal surgery in 2015, and will most likely undergo a follow-up surgery in 2016 to fix a rare complication—unattached abdominal muscles—as a result of her LPAO.

She is a master at seizing every magnificent moment of life and is currently on a journey of self-awareness and discovery. She's beating her wings yet, knowing that someday soon she will be the Phoenix rising from the ashes of all her fears and setbacks.

Want to ride the Juicer train? Best have courage of mind, body, and spirit. Throw off your armor and open your heart. Destination—SOULSDEEP.

You may follow her journey through PAO life at juiceyblogsack.wordpress.com.

Jill Campbell

My PAO Story

About 10 years ago, shortly after I quit playing college soccer in order to have children, I started having pain in my right hip. Over the years, in between having my four wonderful children, I saw orthopedic doctors, chiropractors, physical therapists, and massage therapists. None of the treatment courses brought more than fleeting relief—or even a diagnosis. My husband is in the military, and moving frequently didn't help my progress toward answers, but this year, moving proved to be the best thing that could have happened for me.

Because there isn't a Military Treatment Facility where we are stationed, I was referred to an orthopedic surgeon outside the military system. Upon evaluating my MRI, he referred me to a specialist at Stanford. This is where the divine intervention of this whole journey becomes more clearly evident. The surgeon I was referred to wasn't part of my insurance network, and the original doctor was tasked with finding someone new—someone he had no professional experience with. His medical assistant (who also happened to be a friend from our church) found Dr. Michael Bellino, who I later discovered is a verifiable superstar in the world of hip problems!

After all the waiting games with referrals and insurance, I was excited at the prospect of potentially finding an answer. At the appointment on June 12, it took Dr. Bellino thirty seconds to order a new set of X-rays and another thirty seconds to look at them, diagnose me with hip dysplasia, and explain what it would take to fix it. I should have taken that as a sign; the rest of the process moved nearly as quickly! My husband's job situation was such that he had time off from June 20 to July 13, and then he would be completely unable to take time off for the next 18 months. Not only were there the responsibilities of caring for four young children, but we were also moving at the end of July. I couldn't do this without help! I called Rachel to schedule the surgery and explained the timing of our situation, and she said, "We normally can't schedule surgeries sooner than three months out because Dr. Bellino is so booked up, but just an hour ago someone canceled an appointment on July 2." I was in mild shock, but I knew it was another miracle!

We squeezed in a summer camping trip from June 21-30 in order to give our kids the summer vacation they deserved. My husband also learned that his course wouldn't start until July 23, giving him 10 more days at home. Another miracle. We came home from vacation, did some laundry, arranged child care for the day of surgery, and off we went, leaving an amazing friend with four kids and a grocery list! Because things were so rushed, I had my last pre-op appointment the day before surgery and spent the night at a cousin's house in San Jose while she went down to relieve my friend and stay overnight with the kids. The day came, and despite my fears, I knew we were in the palm of God's hand, or things wouldn't be working out so amazingly smoothly.

There is a hymn that has carried me through countless nerve-wracking experiences in my life:

Lead Kindly Light

1. Lead, kindly Light, amid th'encircling gloom;
Lead Thou me on!
The night is dark, and I am far from home;
Lead Thou me on!
Keep Thou my feet; I do not ask to see
The distant scene—one step enough for me.
2. I was not ever thus, nor pray'd that Thou
Shouldst lead me on.
I loved to choose and see my path; but now,
Lead Thou me on!
I loved the garish day, and, spite of fears,
Pride ruled my will. Remember not past years.
3. So long Thy pow'r hath blest me, sure it still
Will lead me on
O'er moor and fen, o'er crag and torrent, till
The night is gone.
And with the morn those angel faces smile,
Which I have loved long since, and lost awhile!
Text: John Henry Newman, 1801-1890
Music: John B. Dykes, 1823-1876

The next week was a blur; I experienced severe blood loss, consistently low blood pressure, severe nausea, overall weakness, and lethargy. I therefore had no way to regain my strength. I had no choice but to completely trust. I trusted the nurses and CNAs to care for me, which they did wonderfully. I trusted my husband to be there at the hospital with me when he could, and I trusted my cousin and our friends to care for the kids while he was gone. I trusted my body to heal—no small feat considering what it had been put through. Things slowly improved, and I left the hospital six days post-op. Crazy impossibilities followed by little, tender mercy miracles continued to fill every day. The morning after I got home, I fainted. My husband caught me, and no harm was done—another miracle and more proof that I was completely dependent, a state I have never been comfortable with. For the next two weeks, we had constant help from friends, and my dad was able to fly in to help with the kids and packing the house! My husband went back to work, and we moved two days later, with my dad working harder than I've ever seen him work. I was amazed and absolutely humbled.

After only living in the area for a year, we were humbled even more by the constant service and outpouring of love from our friends and neighbors. We moved across town, and the help never stopped. My dad left and my sister-in-law replaced him, nearly passing each other mid-air to and from our hometown. My cousin came down when she could, even taking my girls school shopping. A new member of our church group—whom I'd never even officially met—came to our house to give back-to-school haircuts. People ran errands and brought meals and cleaned our old house and unpacked boxes and took the kids to the park and on and on and on. My extended family had a trip to Yosemite planned, and since my husband couldn't go, I depended on them to help take care of my kids and me. My brother even pushed me in a wheelchair, so I could still enjoy the scenery after I wore myself out. My mom was the fourth family member to come from out of town to stay with us, putting her in "paid time off debt" at work in order to come.

I finally hit that elusive eight-week post-op mark just last Friday, and I am still overwhelmed by the help: offers from multiple friends who were willing to spend a whole day driving me to Stanford and back, offers to watch my kids, rides for the kids to and from school, rides to church, rides everywhere because I can't drive yet! The summer hasn't slowed down any, and we even had two exchange students arrive from Japan yesterday. I'm still on crutches but am blown away by the progress I've made over the last two months, and to think back on all the hours and hours of service it's taken to get us to this point. God is good, and I'm okay with break-neck speed, as long as it's not break-hip speed!! Bring it on. I'm so excited to be able to run, play soccer, ride bikes, and enjoy life with my family pain-free!

About Jill

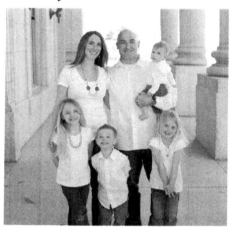

Jill is a 31-year-old mother of four and former (small-time) college soccer player. She lives with her family on the central California coast, though they're originally from Salt Lake City. She loves to travel and will be living abroad in China soon, so being pain-free is an exciting goal!

Annie Bakken Swanberg

The Leap of Faith

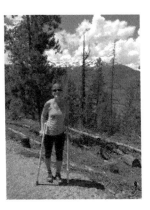

Faith is a funny thing. I wasn't raised with any sort of religious faith; both my parents are scientists, so the very idea of believing and trusting in anything that I can't see with my own eyes has always been foreign to me. Trust, I get. I trust my husband. I trust that going back to school will turn out to have been a worthwhile investment. More to the point of this essay, I trust my surgeon. But faith? I have a hard time with that one. When I was faced with the decision of whether to proceed with a PAO, though, I *had* to find faith, because it was going to be a long, long time until I could know whether I'd made the right decision.

A lot of people who get PAOs are in debilitating pain for years before getting a correct diagnosis, and as soon as they can comfortably ditch the crutches, they can say the surgery has given them their lives back. I was diagnosed very early, which in most ways was a blessing – no one *wants* years of debilitating pain, but it meant there was and is a lot of uncertainty. When I went to my primary sports medicine doctor and said, "Hey, I've had this tendinitis thing going on for a couple months. How do I make it go away?" the last thing I expected to be told was that I needed to have my whole pelvis and femur cut up and rearranged. The surgery was so drastic, and, really, I was fine, wasn't I? Sure, I had to cut some of my runs short because I was limping, but other days I could go for miles and miles without pain. I ran a *marathon* eleven days after my diagnosis. I had occasional random stabbing pain when I pivoted, sometimes when I walked, and as the summer went on, the occasional ache in the joint progressed to being full time. If I sat in one position for too long, I'd limp for the first couple steps after I got up. But if I'd been told to just live with it, I would have been okay with that. The scope of the surgery was entirely out of line with the scope of the symptoms.

However – and here's where being raised by scientist parents comes in, over the course of that summer, I absolutely buried myself in the research literature. I have probably read every paper ever published on the subject of hip dysplasia by now. One thing was undeniable: if I kept running marathons on these shallow hips and twisted femurs, I was going to wind up with hip replacements sooner rather than later. Inside the joint there was already a full-thickness cartilage flap, which was essentially a ticking time bomb. For me, this meant there were much stronger reasons to have the surgery than mere symptom relief. Other things were considerably less clear. The surgery was meant to redistribute the load bearing in my hip, so that the cartilage wear pattern would be different, theoretically slowing the cartilage loss and postponing the onset of osteoarthritis. But PAOs are relatively new, so there is zero literature showing how they actually hold up over fifty years. There is also very little literature regarding whether a PAO can keep an athlete (even a mediocre one like me) performing at her original level. If the data were there, I'd have something to trust. But it isn't there. That's where faith comes in.

It's hard to find stories of people who had a PAO when their symptoms were still relatively mild. We're out there, but I think most folks prefer to avoid surgery at all costs, and the decision-making process is different when you're just trying to get your life back. Deciding to go forward with the surgery when I was still so functional required that I accept some central tenets: 1) that my hip would continue to degenerate; 2) that by the time my pain was bad enough that I *wanted* surgery, it would be too late, because my already-damaged cartilage would be too far gone for a PAO to work; and 3) that a hip replacement would mean the end of my athletic aspirations. It took several months of agonizing – *what if I quit running and switched to cycling as my primary sport? What if the literature and all these doctors I've been consulting are wrong and this won't happen? Where is a crystal ball when I need one?* But I came to accept that these things were true. *I know how this turns out if I don't have the surgery. But… how does it turn out if I do?* There was no way to know. Hence, faith.

My email to my surgeon, on the day I made that leap of faith, reads "All right, let's do this. Terrified though I am, it doesn't do me any good to sit around and wait for it to get worse." I had my PAO in

March of 2015, as well as arthroscopic labral repair *and* a derotational femoral osteotomy to cut my femur in half, twist it back to the proper position, and nail it in place. (As my physical therapist said the other day, "You really got the hammer taken to you.") It's been a long road back, and five months post-op, I'm still running on faith. I can walk pain-free. I'm on my feet all day at work without even thinking about my hip. I can mountain bike. I can pivot around all I want without random stabbing or catching sensations. That deep, constant ache in the joint is long gone. I can hike steep, rocky terrain for two and a half hours so far, and every time I hike, I can go further before my still-atrophied hip muscles start aching. Clearly, my surgeon did a bang-up job, and most people would consider me a success story already. But it's too soon to know whether I'll be able to run trail marathons again, and to me that means it's still too soon to know whether I was right to have the surgery.

And even if I do get back to distance running, the long-term outcome will stay unknown. Maybe on my sixtieth birthday, if my hips are still good, I can say for certain that the PAO was 100% worth it. But maybe I'll still wonder. Without that crystal ball, there's no way of knowing how long my hip really would have held out without surgery. At the same time, there's no point in looking back or dwelling on the unknowable. I choose to believe that I made the right decision. That's all I can do. I already took the leap; now for the rest of my life I will keep facing forward, believing in my decision, keeping the faith.

About Annie

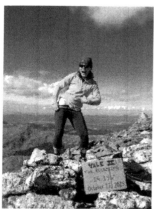

Annie is a 35-year-old grad student living in Boulder, Colorado, arguably the trail-running capital of America. She ran a 50K trail race at just over a year post-op and is now pretty confident that the surgery was worth it.

Jen Lesea-Ames

Lists

Below is my PAO packing list for the hospital and the equipment I used for recovery. If you are having PAO surgery soon, I hope you find these lists useful. Please know that you will not be feeling like doing much while you are in the hospital, so it's best to leave crafty items at home. Also, it's a good idea to leave valuables at home (jewelry, computers—I used my phone for Internet/email).

Packing list for surgery and hospital stay

- ✓ Photo ID and insurance card
- ✓ Toiletries: favorite facial cleansing wipes, favorite lotion, lip balm, deodorant, hair brush, disposable toothbrushes
- ✓ Hat (wear from hospital)
- ✓ Shirt and loose PJ pants (wear to/from hospital)
- ✓ Slip on shoes with a good sole (wear to/from hospital)
- ✓ MP3 player or iPhone for music, headphones and charger
- ✓ Cell phone and charger
- ✓ Eye mask and earplugs
- ✓ Throat lozenges (throat may be sore after breathing tube)
- ✓ Crutches and walker
- ✓ Bag to carry everything
- ✓ A nice comfy, soft blanket (hospital blankets can be scratchy)
- ✓ Stuffed animal for snuggling (my sister bought me a little stuffed cat, and the tag said "Ganz" [think Ganz osteotomy], haha! This is optional, but I found it nice to snuggle with something when I was alone.)

Useful Items For Home Recovery

I bought most of these items on Amazon. Check on the PAO Facebook group to see if other PAO patients may have items for you to borrow or buy used. Also, check with a local medical supply store or local VFW, Elks Club, or thrift store.

✓ Crutches (different styles vary; I was a fan of the Mobileg Ultra crutches.)
✓ Walker with basket (I used the walker for indoor use, crutches for outdoor use, though everyone may vary on usage.)
✓ Shower chair (I used the one without a seat back; different styles vary and depend on personal preference.)
✓ Long-handled sponge for bathing
✓ Elevated toilet seat
✓ "Reacher" device
✓ Leg lift device
✓ Tray table to use for meals in bed
✓ Water bottle with screw-on lid
✓ Ice packs
✓ Lots of pillows for support in bed and while sleeping
✓ Elevated leg rest pillow
✓ "Forever Comfy" seat cushion (I used this when sitting on a hard wooden chair and on the flight home.)

About Jen

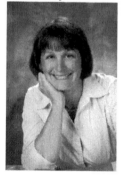

Jen lives her life with a passion to make a positive impact in this world. She is an exercise physiologist by training, a metal-smith jewelry artist, and a former triathlete. Diagnosed at the age of thirty-nine with bilateral hip dysplasia, she had two PAOs in 2014 with Dr. Michael Bellino at Stanford Hospital and Clinics. She is currently enjoying a pain-free life, and it's her mission to help increase awareness of hip dysplasia and PAO surgery by sharing our journeys.

Chapter Four
Recovering from PAO Surgery

"Just keep swimming, just keep swimming…"
Dory, *Finding Nemo*

Editor's Note

Recovering from PAO Surgery

Recovery from PAO surgery varies greatly among patients, lasting from months to years. The rate of recovery depends on a multitude of factors, including, but not limited to, health and fitness level of patient (e.g. smokers have delayed bone growth, and some surgeons will not operate on a smoker unless she has quit at least eight weeks prior to surgery), surgeon experience, care in hospital (which includes pain management), physical therapy protocol, mental attitude of patient, quality of food intake during recovery, and support system (see Chapter Three for Gregory Lammers' caretaker story).

In this chapter, we explore just how individual PAO recovery is amongst patients. The first story is a useful guide to help one battle the feeling of depression, which is a common side effect of PAO surgery recovery. Kelliann Gomez gives practical tips on how to battle depression. Dayna Rose describes what was the longest summer of her life, which entailed five hip surgeries. Her strength and resilience is apparent in her narrative. Cammie Smith explains how she finds inspiration to continue to persevere after a serious car accident set her back in her recovery from her PAO. Ashley Spalla's narrative portrays what can happen when a surgeon not trained to do PAO surgery and the importance of finding a surgeon that is experienced and trained in this hip preservation surgery. Macky Mahrun shares her experience with foot drop, a complication that can occur from PAO surgery. Despite her struggle, she also tries to see the positive aspects in her life.

Amy Lundstedt reflects on the lessons she learned from her PAO and DFO surgery, finding the blessing that this recovery has given her. Katie Di Vitantonio explains how her hip pain and recovery will not define her. Lydia Abell describes the lessons she has learned from her surgery and how she can apply those lessons in her nursing career. Sarah Constantine goes into detail about her second PAO recovery and compares it to her first. Lastly, Sue Gombis' "100 Days" explains the importance of appreciating the little things in life, despite her long road of PAO recovery.

I hope you read each of these stories with an appreciation for the vast differences in PAO recovery. One common thread is apparent: each one has expressed the lessons during this life-changing experience.

Kelliann Gomez

Hippy Self-Care Guide: Considerations to Help You Persevere And Overcome

1. Are you drinking enough water and eating enough nutritional food?

If not, have a glass of water and/or a healthy snack or meal with lots of protein for bone health, like bone broth soup, a kale salad, or raw almonds.

2. Have you said something nice today?

If not, do so. Whether it's in person or online, give someone a genuine compliment or send them a thank-you note telling him/her how awesome he/she is.

3. Have you gotten any exercise today?

If not, try some of your PT exercises, even if it's just ankle pumps or isometrics. Go for a walk/crutch/roll, even if it's just around your house. Better yet, if it's sunny out, soak up some sun, even if that just means just sitting outside or opening a window while you squeeze your glutes.

4. Have you listened to your favorite music lately?

If not, pop on some something good. Sing along; dance in your chair or around the room, etc.… Whatever feels best without hurting you or breaking your restrictions. You can head bob and do jazz hands like a pro!

5. If possible, have you showered recently?

If you haven't, take a shower. If you can't, try something like a sponge bath or even just washing your face and/or hair with your favorite at-home spa products like a mud mask and your favorite aromatherapy.

6. If it's daytime, are you dressed?

If not, put on a nice, clean outfit—something that makes you happy, like a cute shirt or a pretty dress. Even if you aren't able to go out today, it may help you feel more human and put together. If you can't put on or wear your favorite outfit, try cute but comfy clothes like dresses or leggings.

7. If it's nighttime, are you resisting going to sleep or just can't sleep?

Get comfortable in some soft pajamas and blankets in bed. Avoid electronic screens and put on some soothing audio or visualization exercises to help you relax. If you still can't sleep, feel free to get up and try again later, maybe after a cup of chamomile tea or a good book. Poor sleep can most definitely affect mood, so be kind to you and try to rest as much as possible.

8. Have you cuddled a living being recently?

If not, get some cuddles! Ask a loved one for a hug or get some cuddles in with your fur baby. You're worth it, and you're not imposing by asking.

9. Do you feel unattractive?

Take a selfie in the cute outfit you're wearing whether it be the comfy PJs you just put on or the cute outfit, and let people tell you how good you look and how awesome you are by posting it. Bonus: All of that work you put into getting dressed isn't for naught!

If you're self-conscious about your scar, take a scar selfie and show your fellow hippies. We love scars, and we'll remind you just how awesome that warrior wound is!

10. Do you feel ineffective?

Pause and get something done no matter how small. Reply to an email, send someone a thank-you note, do your PT exercises, write a to-do list, etc.… It doesn't have to be big, and it shouldn't be more than you can reasonably do with your pain and/or restrictions.

11. Do you feel inadequate or like you're behind your peers?

Write down a list of accomplishments whether big or small, and remember that your situation and your body are unique. Nobody else's accomplishments detract from your own. Your friend's marathon is impressive, but so is the fact that you got out of bed today with your pelvis all sawed apart.

12. Have you been overexerting yourself mentally, physically, or emotionally lately?

If so, the effects from overexerting yourself can last for days. Give yourself a break with some alone time, physically resting, doing something you enjoy, or trying out a new hobby.

13. Have you recently changed any of your medications in the past few weeks, including skipped doses, changing to generics, and removing medications?

This could be affecting your body in a number of ways. Give things a few days, and then consult with your doctor if symptoms persist.

14. Has your low mood been an ongoing issue?

If not, give yourself a week. Sometimes our perception is skewed, especially between the pain, lifestyle changes, and all of the other facets of hip dysplasia and physical illness. Starting a journal to track your mood and daily obstacles may help.

If this is an ongoing issue, there is no shame in seeking help. You are going through an incredibly trying time, and everybody needs help sometimes.

15. Do you feel bogged down by negativity?

A daily gratitude journal or something similar in which you reflect on what you're thankful for can be uplifting and have a very positive impact on your mood. Save your entries so that you can look back on them later on particularly low days.

You have made it through a lot, and you can make it through this. You are stronger than you realize. Keep going, PAO Warrior!

This guide was adapted from Eponis | Sinope on Tumblr.[3]

About Kelliann

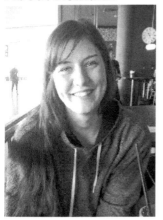

Kelliann was born and raised in the Los Angeles area, but home is wherever her husband and two cats are. She has yet to meet a cat, library, or thrift store that she does not like. Little else has had quite the impact on her life than hip dysplasia has, but for the life lessons she has learned (and is still learning) throughout this journey, she chooses to be grateful. She aspires to continue learning, growing, and experiencing life through the ups, downs, and everything in-between.

Dayna Rose

Persevere and Overcome:
My Surgical Experience

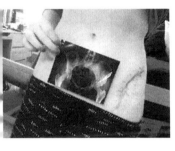

Warrior (noun): a brave or experienced soldier or fighter. See also: an individual who has undergone periacetabular osteotomy.

This self-proclaimed definition does not even begin to describe the way I feel after the longest summer of my life! I am a generally healthy person but have had hip pain since high school. After years of complaining about my hips hurting and being diagnosed as "lazy" by my primary care provider, I finally decided to listen to my body. I had already had one minor hip surgery and loved the entire experience. After researching, I decided that a PAO was the necessary barrier between a total hip replacement and me. Surely, a periacetabular osteotomy would simply be another notch in my belt, right?

My surgeon-to-be, who traveled to Switzerland to learn the Ganz osteotomy from the legend himself, informed me, "This will not be a cute scar." (I love scars, so this did not intimidate me.) "This is the most painful and toughest recovery of all orthopedic surgeries we perform at Children's Hospital," he added nonchalantly. This did not quite register with me, as I still had my head in the clouds. I hurriedly scheduled my PAO for two weeks from that date, ready to endure this surgery and get back to college in time for the fall semester.

The day of my surgery finally came. I often replay this day through my mind over and over, like a broken record. It will always be a vivid memory; I can recall smells, tastes, sensations, and thoughts during the process as if I were experiencing them at this moment. While I confidently waited to get my hip signed by my surgeon and instructions from the anesthesiologist, my mom and dad took turns fidgeting, visiting the restroom to dry-heave, and anxiously sitting in silence. I signed waivers allowing blood transfusions, acknowledging the possibility of infection—the works.

I was wheeled back to anesthesia, past a wall with penguins painted all over it. I was first given nitrous oxide to relax me while they placed an IV and epidural in my back. I remember very vividly becoming very lightheaded all at once; the room swirled around me, and I had extreme difficulty speaking (although I did successfully respond to a knock-knock joke from my anesthesiologist). I recall laughing so hard that the team of anesthesiologists and nurses had to stop and remind me to be still! After the IVs were placed, I became lucid again all at once when they removed the mask. After this, I was wheeled back to the operating room, where they lifted me onto the surgical table while I was still awake (what a strange feeling—as if I was a cadaver on a table ready to be studied). I took in my surroundings and all of the machinery as quickly as I could, knowing it would be my last look.

The very next thing I remember is waking up in the intensive care unit with an oxygen tube down my throat and taped over my mouth. What a wakeup call. I could not open my eyes or respond verbally to the doctors, but I heard my parents' voices. My mom left the room, unable to bear seeing me in such a state. My dad stayed with me and asked me a few questions, to which I simply nodded sluggishly. I became very ill, and it felt like an eternity waiting for the doctors to remove the oxygen tube from my airway.

Later that night, I learned that in surgery, when my surgeon made the initial cut to my pelvic bone, I lost almost half of the blood in my body within 10 minutes' time. My blood pressure was dangerously low, and I had to receive two blood transfusions. After one night in the ICU, I was transferred to a regular room. The rest of the week in the hospital, however, went smoothly (as smoothly as a PAO recovery can go, at least).

The trip home was painful, and the crutch walk into the house was even worse. I slipped and fell coming home, and I broke down and cried for the first time since surgery. I was so frustrated that I couldn't use the bathroom, bathe, or leave the bed without assistance. Other than the typical "had to rely on everyone around me" situation, though, recovery was going well, or so I thought.

Three weeks post-op, I got violently sick, vomiting all night, shaking and sweating with a temperature of 105 degrees. After a few nights of hoping it was just the flu, I went to the emergency department. Sure enough, I had an infection. I was admitted and got two more surgeries to clean out the infected area. I also received a PICC line, an IV that was placed into my arm and went close to my heart in order to administer antibiotics three times daily. I was at the hospital for a week and finally was allowed to go home.

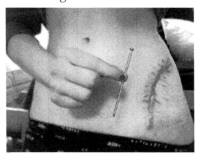

Another three weeks later, my incision (which was supposed to stop draining after three days) was still draining! Again, I was admitted into the hospital for two more surgeries. During the first surgery of this stay, the surgeons and fellows had realized that the infection had spread into my hip bone. They removed my screws about 10 months early and put in a vacuum dressing, which functioned to "suck out" all the infection and blood and stimulate tissue healing. To cut down the number of surgeries and trauma to my body, the team decided to change my vacuum dressing in my room while I was wide awake (yikes!). It was a nerve-wracking situation, having a full team of doctors surrounding me and speaking in medical jargon. My fifth and final surgery (for now) was just a repeat of the others, and felt like a repeat, too (I cursed at the sight of the dreaded penguin wall every time); the anesthesiologists lazily reminded me of the risks, I listlessly signed waivers, and I again drifted off to sleep. This time, my iliac crest was shaved down in order to close my tissue over the bone.

After this surgery, it took nearly two months for my incision to heal up! I finally got my PICC line removed, and I started school again on time. I started walking on my own just one week before heading back to campus! Now, my scar is very deformed and looks more like a concave trench than scar tissue, and I have been advised to get plastic surgery to correct it. However, I love my scar, and I would hate to throw away the visual representation of the strength I gained this summer. It is truly a humbling experience to walk around day-to-day and think, "I can walk!" and smile to myself. This dreadful experience has led me to a positive light, always grateful that things did not go worse. If there is one lesson to take from this story, it is this: don't take anything for granted, *especially* your hip joints; those things are so crucial to everyday movement and activity! Every day I look at my scar, and it represents my conquest of physical and mental pain, a reminder of what I am capable of enduring, and a beacon of hope. My advice to current and future PAO participants is from the wise Winston Churchill: "If you're going through hell, keep going."

About Dayna

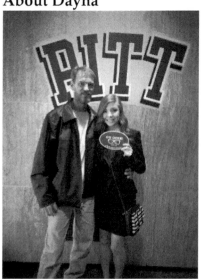

Dayna, a 20-year-old college student at the University of Pittsburgh, aspires to become a mortician after she graduates. She has had six hip surgeries now (five just this summer!) and loves to share her scar and story.

Cammie Smith

Consider It All Joy

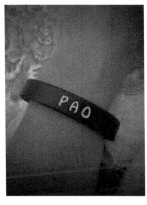

So, here I am, five-and-a-half months after surgery, and still in pain—pain significant enough that tomorrow is my last day of work for a little while. I tried my best to return to my job as a high school English teacher, but my body just isn't ready. The original plan was that I would have returned to work off crutches and off most of the medications I am still currently taking. However, after my car accident in July (a girl T-boned me going forty-five miles per hour, completely totaled my car, and I sustained injuries to my neck, back, and recovering hip), I am significantly behind in my recovery. I've done my best to attempt to ditch the crutches and ditch the medicine since returning to work; neither attempt has been successful. Dr. Olson and I talked last week and decided it would be best if I fully concentrate on my rehabilitation right now, at least until I can get off of crutches and hopefully stop taking so much medication. It was a very hard decision because going back to work has been such an emotional boost for me; those emotional boosts are so incredibly important when riding the roller coaster of PAO recovery.

Unfortunately, though, I have plateaued in my rehab at this point. Physical therapy decreases my pain to a certain extent, and then I return to work, and the pain escalates to the point that if I don't take medication, I can't function. So, here we are. I'm still on crutches, still on medication, and still have a leg with the majority of my muscle groups stuck in contraction (seriously, you name it, it's contracted!). There's a difference at this point, though. See, I slammed into the wall of hopelessness and depression when I had my car wreck. That setback, coupled with Valium for the muscle spasms, sent this already sensitive soul spiraling into a deep, dark depression. But I recognized the symptoms, came off of the Valium, and scratched my way out of that darkness. Now, I feel stronger, mentally and emotionally. At this point, I have reclaimed my lost, fierce desire to be healthy. At this point, I am starting to catch glimpses of a light at the end of this incredibly long tunnel. The PAO Warrior in me has reclaimed her spirit. For the next four to five weeks, my sole purpose in life is to strengthen my leg and hip enough so that I can walk without crutches for an entire day, pain-free (which hopefully will naturally lend itself to a significant decrease in my medication usage). Challenge accepted!

And now for the title connection, the "Ah ha!" moment, the "I hear you, God" realization. It's been a rough week in the parenting department. Heck, it's been a rough three years in the parenting department! Starting with my early symptoms, spanning through a pregnancy/delivery, two surgeries, and now PAO recovery, parenting has been more along the lines of "do whatever keeps the peace" rather than raise well-behaved, good little listeners. I could write a whole dissertation entitled "The Struggles of Parenting through Chronic Pain," but I'll save that for my next degree. Ha! Anyway, we are currently trying to re-train our little people to be good listeners, share, behave at school, etc. It is the third week of school, and our six-year-old has already gotten in trouble at school twice for talking too much and interrupting during class (poor kid...I really do think there is a valid argument that it's genetic). Avery came home "on orange" today for getting in trouble talking and interrupting.

We are having the same problem at home, as well as some issues with her testing the limits to see how far she can push us. Last week, her consequence was to lose the iPad, TV, and after-dinner treat, and she had an early bedtime. Clearly, losing all of those privileges must have been a joke to her, because here we are exactly seven days later, and she's on orange, which is worse than the on yellow from last week! To top it all off, within half an hour of getting home, she spills milk all over the kitchen floor after being told by her father to wait for help and screams her way up the stairs into her bedroom, blaming her little sister (who is two, for the record) for making her get the glass of milk. She did this knowing she is already going to lose privileges because of her behavior at school! Ugh! Needless to say at this point, we've got to drop the hammer. This time we made the consequences fit the action. Avery could not be quiet and refrain from interrupting at school, so we made her do so at home. She had to stay in her bedroom the entire evening, with no toys and no electronic devices (only books), until bedtime. It is probably too early to tell, but based on her behavior the past three hours, I think solitary confinement might be the answer to our parenting prayers. It breaks my heart, but she has cried and been more affected by this consequence than anything else we have tried thus far. I suppose time with tell.

While Avery has spent the last three hours crying or staring at the ceiling in her room (she refuses to read), I have started reading a book I bought several months ago called *Boundaries with Kids* by Dr. Henry Cloud and Dr. John Townsend. I know, I'm a dork; I'll own it. We English teacher-types always look to books to help us understand the world around us and the things we cannot control. I get to the chapter called "Pain Can Be a Gift," and I have this enlightening experience. The book says, "Lesson number one in parenting and in life is 'Growth involves pain.'" As I'm reading this chapter, I realize that so much of my parenting struggles are due to the fact that I don't want my girls to experience pain, and when they seem to be in pain, it breaks my heart (e.g. Avery lying in her bed crying right now because, in her words, she's lonely). I have been through excruciating pain the past three years. I don't want my girls to experience pain, be it mental or physical. But if I want to raise well-rounded children who can handle the struggles life can and will throw at them, they have to learn to cope with pain and difficulties, even in the form of consequences for their actions. As I continue reading, I come to the second section entitled "Consider It All Joy," and this is when the light bulb moment happens! Here is the beginning of the section, word for word:

"The following passage from the Book of James is one of my favorites: 'Consider it pure joy, my brothers, whenever you face trials of many kinds, because you know that the testing of your faith develops perseverance. Perseverance must finish its work so that you may be mature and complete, not lacking anything' (James 1:2-4)." Wow. Just wow. This excerpt took me very quickly from "Parent with a disobedient child" mode to "Child of God who needs to see the bigger picture" mode. Why is this passage so impactful, you ask? See my pictures: the bracelet that I wear and have worn on my wrist from the moment I received it shortly after my surgery has the acronym for my surgery, PAO, on one side, and three words on the other side, the words that a fellow PAO patient chose to represent those of us who have "made it to the other side" with this surgery and the corresponding recovery. Those words are Persevere and Overcome. Sweet Lisbeth Kish sends each PAO Warrior one of these bracelets,

upon request, as a symbolic everyday reminder of what we have been through and what we are capable of. So, a week-and-a-half ago, I received my gift from Lisbeth with the quote "It's not the destination, but the journey that matters most," and this week I come across the verse "Perseverance must finish its work so that you may be mature and complete, not lacking anything." I don't think this message could be any louder or any clearer. As my Uncle Jeff says, "Bravo, God! Bravo!"

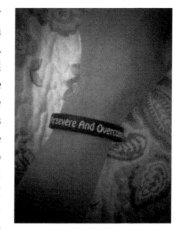

And so, with my fierce desire to be healthy, and doing my best to "consider it all joy," I will keep striving to persevere and overcome as my PAO journey continues....

About Cammie

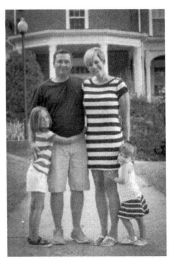

Cammie Smith is a 36-year-old wife, mother, and high school teacher who strives daily to keep God first in all she says and does. She loves reading, shopping, and Reese's peanut butter anything. Cammie played softball and danced for the majority of her early years up through high school, and she never had problems with her hips until recently.

Her dysplasia was not diagnosed until she was 34, after breaking her foot and walking in a cast for five-and-a-half months while pregnant. She had a right PAO on April 22, 2015, at Duke Regional Hospital with Dr. Steven Olson. As she continues along the road of PAO recovery, her goal is simple: to persevere and overcome during this challenging stage of her life in the hopes of one day being pain-free.

Ashley Spalla

My Story Has Only Begun...

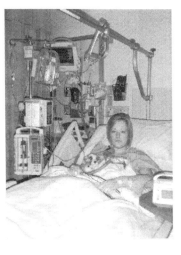

For as long as I can remember, I have been an athlete. I grew up doing gymnastics, playing softball and basketball, running, and participating in competitive cheerleading in high school. Being an athlete was part of my identity. When I went off to college to study biology and pursue a career in medicine, I used running as a form of therapy. Being active was a normal part of my day, just like eating or taking a shower. I was also familiar with the injuries that came with an active lifestyle. I had always pushed myself both physically and mentally.

I wanted to take my abilities to the next level, so my sophomore year of college I enlisted in the Army and joined ROTC. I spent that summer at Basic Combat Training (BCT) and Advanced Individual Training (AIT). In the fall, I continued my Army training through ROTC to become a U.S. Army officer. During the winter of 2008-2009, I decided to join our intramural ROTC basketball team for fun. Our ROTC teams played in a tournament at the University of Notre Dame in January 2009. My body and hips were sore, but nothing I didn't chalk up to training. The tournament was rough physically, and I had stabbing and searing pain through my right hip. I tried giving my hip time to recover, but it made no difference.

I knew something was not right with my hip and decided to go to my sports doctor. At most, I thought I tore cartilage and would need my hip scoped, but little did I know that torn cartilage would be the least of my problems. I had an immediate MRI, and within twenty-four hours my doctor called me back with the results. I knew with that quick of a response, the news was not going to be good. He told me I had a torn labrum, labral cyst, soft tissue tears, and hip dysplasia. "Hip dysplasia?" I replied, "Like a German shepherd?" He also told me that this is something that will require surgical intervention and referred me to a hip specialist. The hip specialist told me that treating hip dysplasia is much more specialized and is not something he does and only a handful of surgeons treat. I was also told that I was fortunate because there was a local hip surgeon in Indianapolis who could correct the dysplasia.

It took a few weeks to get into this surgeon for a consult. In the meantime, anxiety ran rampant, as did my searches on the Internet. It was not encouraging when the first searches pertained to canine hip dysplasia. There was little information about adult hip dysplasia. No Facebook groups existed; there were no support sites or foundations available to turn to for help. I felt so alone and so angry about my circumstances. The pain and symptoms in my hip deteriorated rapidly. Sleep was difficult and even getting in and out of my car was horribly painful. I felt as if everything I had worked and trained for was in vain.

My consult with the specialist came and went, and surgery was scheduled for the summer. I would have my hip socket broken, rotated, and screwed back into a position that would allow adequate coverage of the femoral head, which would ultimately give me more stability and preserve my joint. No big deal. The pain was getting worse, as was my apprehension about the surgery. Just talking about the surgery made me break down into tears. Depression and anxiety had set in, and I got to the point where I needed help coping. It was at that point when my primary care physician prescribed Prozac to help ease the highs and lows. I tried my best to prep for the surgery by getting items for the hospital and things to help during my recovery.

Surgery day came, and I was a nervous wreck. I did not sleep at all the night before. My parents were able to stay with me while I was being prepped, and while I waited to be wheeled back to the OR, I was able to hold it together until I was taken back to the OR. As soon as I went through the

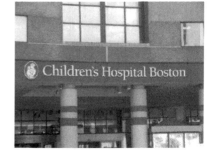

doors and saw multiple surgical tables, tables of equipment, my two surgeons, and a ton of surgical staff, I panicked. I began crying hysterically and hyperventilating. They didn't even bother waiting to put me under until I was transferred and positioned because I was so upset. It's the last thing I remembered until I woke up briefly in PACU, then in my room.

The hospital stay was brutal. It was the first time I ever needed to stay overnight in a hospital. My leg was huge, due to swelling, because no drains were placed. It took weeks for the swelling to even reasonably subside. Pain management was extremely difficult. I did better in PT than I anticipated, but every movement was excruciatingly painful. I couldn't believe what I had gotten myself into, and I wondered if I had made a huge mistake. I spent five nights in the hospital before being discharged to my parents' house. The only time I saw my surgeon was in pre-op and the day I was discharged.

The problems developed immediately post-op. The swelling alone took months to resolve. I also developed nerve pain and issues that would later be diagnosed as CRPS (Chronic Regional Pain Syndrome) and required special medication to help calm the nerves. My surgical incision had some staples, stitches, and glue. It also took nearly three months to completely close and heal. Four to five months post-op, the pain increased, and I had developed stress fractures, despite still needing the aid of crutches to walk. One problem after another arose, and pain never really seemed to go away.

About a little over a year post-op, the pain had not ceased, so my doctor decided to re-scope the hip. My hip actually needed more repairs due to extensive damage following my PAO, when my activity level was minimal, than prior to the PAO, when I was very active. I was frustrated because I thought the entire purpose of the PAO was to prevent this exact issue from occurring. After speaking with some other PAO Warriors and doing some research, I found a research paper that explained the PAO process, failure rates, symptoms of failed PAOs, etc. The physician who created the PAO or Ganz osteotomy, Dr. Reinhold Ganz, conducted the study. My symptoms fit everything listed in the research paper. I was dumbfounded. I could not believe this was happening. It also meant that completing ROTC and commissioning as an Army officer would not be possible. It was the end of a dream and a reality I was not prepared to face.

I ultimately found out that the surgeon who performed my PAO was not a trained hip preservation specialist, and he did not have the experience he told me that he had. The hip surgeon who referred me at first told me that he was unaware that the doctor was not trained, but when speaking with him at a later date, he told me that he did not inform his patients of other trained surgeons in places such as St. Louis, Detroit, or Boston because he "did not think his patients would want to travel for care." I was furious and devastated that my ability to choose had been taken from me. I was a very angry and resentful person for a long time. I was also deeply hurt that people who should have been looking out for my best interest had violated my trust.

To even begin to fix my hip, I did endless research and decided to see the best. I scheduled an appointment to see Dr. Millis at Boston Children's Hospital. Dr. Millis quickly realized there was more than a botched surgery to overcome. He had me see a geneticist, and I was diagnosed with Ehlers-Danlos syndrome, which is a connective tissue disorder that causes a defect in the collagen and tissues of the body. It causes joint hypermobility, instability, poor healing, delicate skin, and even heart and vascular issues. It was contributing to the myriad of issues I had been enduring but had been overlooked by other doctors as "weird" until Dr. Millis.

I have now been a patient of Dr. Millis for more than five years and have had 21 surgeries total, eight surgeries on my right hip alone. The most recent of surgeries was last year. Surgeries will always be needed for maintenance. I have been a staple at my PT clinic, and my physical therapist has become a friend and supporter as I have endured surgery after surgery.

I started my PAO journey six-and-a-half years ago, and it has forever changed my life. My hip journey is not finite, but I am determined to continue doing what I love and to never let anyone tell me never. This journey has taught me that I am stronger and more capable than I ever could have imagined. It has taken years to come to a place of acceptance and peace with my circumstances, but there are days that I still struggle. This journey has reignited my love for science as well as a desire to raise awareness and further hip dysplasia research.

My story has only begun....

"Hardships often prepare ordinary people
for an extraordinary destiny."
C.S. Lewis

About Ashley

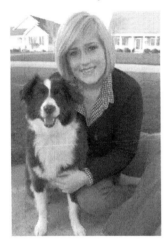

Ashley Spalla, now 27 years old, was 21 years old when she was diagnosed with bilateral hip dysplasia. She never knew she had hip dysplasia and had been a very active child growing up. She continued a high level of activity into college, which included distance running, CrossFit, and Army ROTC. She knew something was wrong after experiencing searing hip pain during an ROTC basketball tournament in January 2009. After an MRI, Ashley was diagnosed with hip dysplasia, labral tears, and ligament tears. She was more than terrified, and the lack of available knowledge only worsened her anxiety and fear.

She had her RPAO in June 2009. During her PAO journey, she was also diagnosed with a rare connective tissue disorder called Ehlers-Danlos syndrome, classic type. Ashley has endured 21 surgeries total: 11 on her hips and eight of these on her right hip. Her right hip has undergone a PAO/scope, arthroscopy, hardware removal/revision, femoral varus rotational osteotomy, trochanteric osteotomy, femoral hardware removal with revision, infection IND, and arthroscopy/hybrid open surgery. Little did she know that this would begin a journey she never could have anticipated.

Macky Maruhn

The Journey That Never Ends

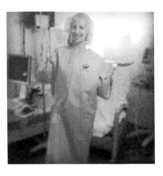

I was just 24 years old when I found out that I had bilateral hip dysplasia. My orthopedic doctor knew exactly what to prescribe for this: a major reconstructive surgery called a periacetabular osteotomy, also known as a PAO. Two days after my 25th birthday, I flew to Oakland, California, from Portland, Oregon, and met my surgeon for the first time. Two days later, I took a cab to the hospital with my mom and grandmother to undergo surgery on my right hip.

When I first woke up, I couldn't move my entire leg. At first, I thought it was because I had gone through a major surgery and my body was in shock. I was hysterical over the pain. A nurse gave me something for the pain, and I was in and out of consciousness for a few hours. Eventually, one of my surgeons came into the recovery room to see how I was doing. He squeezed my right foot as he came around the bed, but I felt nothing. I looked at my foot and tried as hard as I could to make my toes move. Not even a little wiggle. When I explained what I was trying to do but getting no response, my doctor began to test my reflexes and sensory capabilities, but to no avail, my foot was utterly useless.

Once I got settled into a room, someone came in to see how I was feeling and took a look at my foot. I soon learned that my sciatic nerve had been overstretched during the surgery, and I was experiencing foot drop. My doctors were confident that it was just a temporary symptom, and in a few days I would be able to feel and move my foot again. That never happened. During my five-day vacation in the hospital, I struggled with the pain of having a broken hip, learning how to move without putting much weight on it, and how to do everyday tasks with my new limitations. Once I was released, I settled into a swanky boutique hotel right on the bay with my mom and grandmother. Even though I was in an incredible amount of pain, we still tried to make the best of our time there.

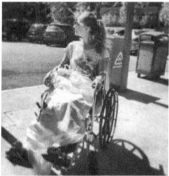

On the day before we were supposed to leave California, I had an ultrasound done on my leg to make sure there weren't any blood clots. My foot had swollen up twice its normal size and turned purple. The poor technician almost got punched in the face because of the pain the ultrasound created. Thankfully, I got the all clear to fly back to Oregon. I had only brought crutches with me, but since I could barely stand upright without being in a ton of pain, let alone maneuver crutches, I had to rely on a walker and wheelchair. I truly felt like I had hit rock bottom. Prior to my PAO, I had been a cheerleader for a minor league football team and had spent most of my middle and high school years dancing, playing basketball, and doing track. Never did I imagine I would be confined to a wheelchair by the time I was 25.

At my six-week checkup, I saw the orthopedic doctor that had first told me about PAOs. Although he had never performed a PAO, he was in constant communication with the surgeon who did the operation so I didn't have to fly back and forth between Oregon and California. The first X-rays I got to see really shocked me. I only needed two screws, but the cuts made in the bones were much larger than I had imagined. Except from a doctor's point of view, it wasn't as bad as it seemed, and there was already new bone growth, so technically I was doing great. If only my pain levels were lower, I might have believed it. I don't know how my mother put up with all of those nights she spent changing out my ice packs, waking me up to take my medication, or just listening to me cry about my situation. Then again, that's what moms are for, right?

It took at least three months for me to feel comfortable enough to ditch my walker and use crutches. By this time I was starting to feel the bottom of my foot and push it down towards the ground, but I still couldn't feel my leg from the knee down on the outer right side or the top of my foot. My nerve specialist did an electromyogram (EMG) to see how my muscles responded to nerve stimulation and confirmed that the sciatic nerve was damaged around my hip. Furthermore, my peroneal nerve was basically dormant, and there was nothing I could do but patiently wait to see if it would wake up again. So, I decided to take matters into my own hands and look for answers. My endless hours of searching on Google gave me little hope. The likeliness of waking up with foot drop after a PAO is very rare. Those who do usually fully recover within a year. I was quickly learning my trial was unique, and I wouldn't find the answers I was looking for on an Internet search. I did, however, find a fantastic PAO group on Facebook full of fierce hip warriors from all across the world. Through them, I found inspiration to keep pushing forward one step at a time. I was also directed to look into getting a specific brace so that I could walk somewhat normally again.

Soon after finding out about Allard USA's ToeOFF brace, I was in an office getting fitted for one. The day I picked up my brace, I felt like I was getting my life back. September 12, 2015, will be the two-year anniversary of my PAO. I still cannot lift my foot up, but I am hopeful that the small muscle movements only I can feel mean one day I will be able to move my foot visibly. Since my gait is abnormal, I've developed bursitis in my right hip, and my SI joints shift differently. I'm in pain 24/7, either because the nerve pain is flaring up or because my hip is yelling at me. My left hip is beginning to give me pain more often, and I'm doing all that I can to hold off on surgery. Sleeping on my right side is simply out of the question, and long car rides are rough. The worst part about all of this is not being able to wear all of the heels, flats, and flip-flops I have in my closet. I'm stuck wearing sneakers daily.

Since my surgery, I've learned to celebrate small victories no matter what. As time has gone by, I have been able to wear certain types of heels without a brace and go on hikes, even though I never thought I'd hike again. I can push through the pain and work 40 hours per week all while on my feet. And I can drive! My journey through recovery has been a long one and nothing like I had envisioned. There are days when I pray that I could rewind time and change my decision to have a PAO. There are days when I feel as if I can conquer the world and am genuinely grateful to have been chosen for this particular trial.

Most of all, this experience has reminded me to look for the rainbow in the rain and to never give up hope. It has shown me how strong and resilient I truly am, and it's given me so many beautiful friendships with people I wouldn't have met otherwise. I am a true PAO Warrior, and that makes my life extra special!

About Macky

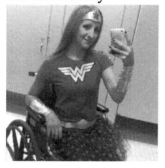

Macky Maruhn is a 26-year-old crazy cat lady who jokingly refers to herself as the cripple friend. She enjoys dancing, traveling, and sharing her unique story with others as often as she can. She hopes to inspire others to climb the mountains in their life with as much determination as she has.

"The greater the obstacle, the more glory in overcoming it."
Moliere

Amy Lundstedt

Lessons I've Learned

I found out I had a hip issue in May of 2013. It was not diagnosed as hip dysplasia until March 2015. I had an extremely frustrating two years of not being able to do any of the activities I loved doing. So when I received the news that my problem would take not only a PAO but also a DFO to fix, I was upset. I honestly thought I could just get my hip scoped and then it would be a quick and easy recovery. After the initial shock wore off, I began to count my blessings.

Now, post-surgery, these are the things I am walking away with:

- I have an answer to my problem, finally!
- I have a surgeon I trust in Denver, who has been great.
- The outpouring of love from family and friends both here and from afar has been amazing, and I feel so blessed every day.
- The support of the PAO community has been so wonderful and helpful with questions and concerns. I've made some great friends.
- I can go back to the activities I love with no more hip pain.

The journey for me is only half over. I have to go back and do the other side; however, now I feel ready to tackle this. I am going into it not with fear—but with hope that it will get better and the knowledge that this too shall pass. This set of surgeries is no joke. It truly takes PAO Warriors to make it through. I am thankful for people who understand catheters, shower chairs, sleeping in recliners for weeks/months, handicapped parking, the joys and frustrations of PT, the excitement of every X-ray, and the simple pleasure of walking unassisted.

About Amy

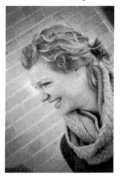

Amy has led a super-active life for the last 33 years. When she was 31, she started having right hip pain, which went undiagnosed for two years. When it was finally diagnosed, she was relieved to be able to do something about it, yet frustrated that it took two years to figure out. She has had multiple friends tell her, "Man, that is hard, and I don't even like doing physical things, so it must be really hard for you." The answer is yes; everything about this is super hard. However, it does get better. Her name is Amy Lundstedt, and she is a PAO Warrior.

Katie Di Vitantonio

Better

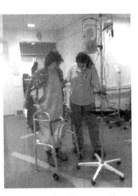

Running that fateful 5K in April 2014 was both a blessing and curse, as it is what put me on the path I am on now. Discovering that my labrum had torn and learning at the same time that I would have to stop running and take a semester off of school to have my hip repaired was devastating, and at times it made me want to scream. I realized with every passing day from that point on—from meeting with Dr. Ernest Sink at the Hospital for Special Surgery's Center for Hip Preservation in October 2014, to having my left hip fixed on March 4, 2015—that all the highs and lows have made me a stronger individual emotionally, mentally, and physically.

March 5, 2015—1 Day Post-Op

I'm still having a difficult recovery: it was incredibly hard waking up in the recovery room, I needed a blood transfusion, I was taken off the morphine drip because of adverse reactions, and I experienced two infections and a stress fracture, and I'm still having some delayed bone growth. But despite it all, there have been plenty of highlights: starting physical therapy and learning to walk normally again, being able to now walk without my crutches, and going on a hike. But above all, with all that this surgery brought about—both positive and negative, the greatest highlight of this ordeal has been having a phenomenal support group: Dr. Sink and his team, my physical therapists at MCRC, all the PAO Warriors on the Periacetabular Osteotomy (PAO) support group on Facebook whose insight and stories have been so helpful, and last but certainly not least is my mom, dad, older brother, and boyfriend.

I can honestly say that without the love, support, and encouragement I have received from everyone, I would not be as far along as I am. I have always had a reservoir of inner strength and determination to fight, but sometimes everyone needs a shoulder to lean on and have some help—no matter how proud or stubborn they are. We're only human, but we are also warriors who have proved that we are unstoppable.

May 21, 2015—2.5 Months Post-Op

I know that I still have a long way to go in terms of my recovery, but I'm determined to keep pushing forward and getting stronger, so I can reach all of my goals and aspirations. My hip dysplasia is not going to define me as an individual, but my actions will. Whenever I get upset or frustrated because I need to use my crutches for a day or two due to being sore, I can put it in perspective by looking back and seeing how far I have come, and that helps more than anything. I have shown myself that I am much stronger than I have ever given myself credit for and that knowledge is one of the best lessons that I've been able to take from having "screwed"-up hips.

> "Only those who will risk going too far
> can possibly find out how far one can go."
> T.S. Eliot

About Katie

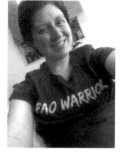

Katie Di Vitantonio is 21 years old and in the process of recovering from her left PAO, which was done on March 4, 2015. She never knew that she had bilateral hip dysplasia; it wasn't ever something that crossed her orthopedic doctor's mind or her own, to be honest. All they knew was that she was loose jointed. It wasn't until she tore her labrum running a charity 5K at her college that she found out she had hip dysplasia and would need to have it corrected. The thought of how violent and invasive this procedure was terrified her, but she knew that it had to be done. Looking back now, four months later, she can really see that she hadn't been living her life to the fullest because she was undiagnosed for so long. It's been a tough road, and she knows it isn't over yet, but she knows she's heading in the right direction and is on the road to getting better.

Lydia Abell

Learning from the Journey of PAO Recovery

"You need bilateral hip replacements." These were the shocking words my doctor told me after I had finally convinced myself to get my strange hip pains looked at by a professional. I remember getting in the car and calling my husband with this news that seemed so out of place for a 29-year-old like me to receive. I went there expecting to get some exercises to help my pain, only to leave with referrals to specialists and the news of impending surgery...an operation I thought only old people needed, and a diagnosis I associated only with newborn babies and dogs. The next few weeks are a bit of a blur, including two visits to two specialists who diagnosed bilateral hip dysplasia secondary to having had Legg-Calve-Perthes disease as a child, which was never diagnosed. It was with my second and third opinions that I learned about the PAO surgery and gained hope in reconstruction and hip preservation.

My husband and I had been trying to have a child for quite some time and had suffered a few pregnancy losses. Upon receiving my diagnosis, I was told by one doctor, "Whatever you do, don't get pregnant because you already have very little cartilage and the weight gain will not be good for you. Ideally you should have surgery in the next six months." Ironically enough, ten days later, we learned we were expecting a baby. Fast forward 14 months later, and there I found myself, going into surgery for my PAO and PFO with my husband and five-month-old baby girl waiting for me on the other side. I now know that our little girl was the perfect gift from God to help me through my recovery. When I wanted to give up or became discouraged, I would see my little girl's face and remember what a miracle gift she was to us, and it gave me motivation to persevere.

It's the recovery that has taught me the most about myself. I have always been the one to look after others. I'm a nurse by profession, and caring for people is what I do best. But this entire situation and recovery process has taught me what true dependence means — dependence on others to help me with simple everyday activities and to help me take care of my daughter when I could not bend down, pick her up, or carry her. I learned what it means to rely on God to help me emotionally and spiritually persevere and find joy and purpose in a slow and painful recovery. I learned that pain is real and physical therapy takes hard work. I learned that PAO really does require us to "persevere and overcome" quite a bit. I learned how important support is from others who have been through or are going through PAO surgeries. I learned how grateful I am to have my amazing husband who so graciously took care of me without ever complaining. And I learned how important friends and family are to a successful recovery.

It is in the post-op phase of this journey that I have discovered so much about myself, about my family and friends, and about my faith. It really is a journey; it is an affliction, a blessing, a hardship, an opportunity, a truly life-changing and mind-altering event. It brought tears of sadness and pain from nerve, muscle, and bone healing, as well as tears of joy when I could at last start walking and especially when I could hold my baby again. It has taught me to be a better nurse because I now know what it means to be in pain and to be stripped of independence, allowing me to now have true empathy for my patients. It has taught me not to take life for granted. It has shown me the importance of kindness, grace, compassion, and help from others. Now that I am able to walk again, I feel inspired to do my best to reciprocate this to others.

This has been my PAO journey. I pray you feel God's blessing and love as you embark on or continue yours.

About Lydia

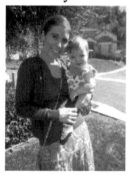

Lydia Abell is 30 years old and lives with her husband and daughter in Santa Cruz, California. She loves the outdoors, exploring new places, and spending time with family and friends. She's worked as an ER nurse the past eight years and loves her job. She sees each day as a gift from God and tries to enjoy life to the fullest.

Sarah Constantine

New and Improved

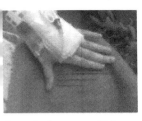 I woke up amidst darkness and confusion. Someone was holding my hand, and a couple other people seemed to be hovering around the curtains. Light escaped into the room under the door and through the blinds. Slowly, memories flood back in: hospital gowns, IVs, nurses, anesthesia... hip surgery!

After a six-hour surgery and hours in the recovery room that I do not remember, I was finally aware and settled in my room on the 3E Wing in Lucille Packard's Children Hospital at Stanford. My mom, girlfriend, and nurses saw my eyes open and began talking. Groggily I tried to keep up with the conversation, but nothing seemed to stick. I was hooked up to an IV, but thirst still seemed to overcome me. One IV was capped, and one was connected to fluids and antibiotics. I was also attached to two catheters. One, the epidural, ran through my spine to provide pain relief, while the other was a Foley catheter to help me urinate. Additionally, I had a plastic tube draining blood and fluids from my incision area and electrodes placed across my chest to track my vitals. Sleep came quickly and easily that night.

The next morning I felt much better; the epidural was doing its job. Nurses had come and gone in the night, checking vitals and making sure I could feel my toes, and they continued to come throughout the morning. I do not recall much that happened in the first few days but according to my family, I talked for hours and wanted to make sure they wrote down everything! As stated by the record, I immediately asked for the epidural in my back to be turned off so I could begin controlling my pain orally, ate breakfast, and had visitors throughout the day.

Each day spent in the hospital was better than the last. I had amazing nurses and an amazing surgeon, Dr. Pun, who checked on me every day. Physical therapists and occupational therapists came each day and always pushed me past my limit. Every day brought different challenges and new things to cry about. The first few times of getting out of bed made me feel like I was going to pass out from pain, but I always seemed to manage. While in the hospital, I even had the wonderful opportunity to connect with another PAO Warrior who was recovering down the hall! It was amazing having the support from another family going through the same struggles as mine at the exact same time.

On day four, I left the hospital in my mother's tiny, secure Prius. We drove four-and-a-half awful hours until we hit the bucket of heat and pollution we call home: Bakersfield. Though it was hot, and the pain meds made me even hotter, I was happy to be home. Now within the comforts of home, I faced new challenges. All of a sudden I had to worry about how to stand up from a couch and how I should maneuver with crutches through a bedroom. Something as simple as going into the other room took a lot of thought. Slowly everything became easier. Moving my leg became second nature to my mom, and helping me get food was now a normal thing for my siblings. Showering proved a little difficult, but after being in the hospital, I had no modesty left.

Now to many of you PAO Warriors out there, this recovery seems simple compared to what you've been through. And admittedly this was my second time experiencing all of this. Six months earlier, I underwent the same surgery on the opposite hip. Recovery the first time did not go as smoothly. I was in the hospital for eight days and never got my pain under control. I was discharged and given instructions for home, but nothing seemed to improve much. I stayed heavily medicated for the following couple of weeks until deciding this was not okay and returning to the hospital. After many blood tests, ultrasounds, X-rays, and MRIs, the array of doctors working with me determined I had a pleural effusion, which had made my lung partially collapse. I was immediately readmitted to the hospital. Fluid was drawn from my back (ouch) and tested for so many diseases I lost count. Eventually the pulmonologist said I was okay to go home and they would call me with the results. A week later, I got a call saying everything was okay and the fluid in the cavity would go away on its own. Even though this was not hip pain, it affected my recovery drastically. I was short of breath constantly and had pain in my rib area every second. Throughout all of this, I was going to physical therapy and attending school at University of California, Santa Cruz. Needless to say, my life was chaotic.

The second time around has gone so much better already, and I foresee the rest of my recovery going even better. Dr. Pun is there every time I feel something might be wrong, and my fabulous physical therapist, Nikki Losee, is about to start helping me strengthen my muscles and roll out my kinks until I cry. I definitely couldn't be taking this journey alone; my mom and girlfriend are always within earshot to help, a wonderful Facebook 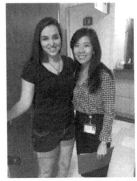 group of pre- and post-PAO Warriors is there any time I have a weird question, all the nurses at Lucille Packard Children's Hospital at Stanford watched over me day and night during my hospital stays, and of course the best surgeon I know, Dr. Pun, gave me new hips for a new pain-free life. All of these people have helped me on my road to recovery.

Learning how to walk again is a weird experience. After progressing from two crutches to one, and then to a cane, it almost feels unreal when you take your first unaided step. Going through this long journey allows you to discover muscles that you never knew could hurt so much, and nerves that run down your whole leg feel like they are on fire when they try to regenerate around your incision. You also learn that bathrooms are in fact not handicap accessible despite the wheelchair sign on the wall, people will drop doors on your face even when you kindly ask them not to, and people will illegally park in handicap spaces despite not being handicapped or having proper documentation to prove it.

Despite all these small yet irritating things, I am incredibly happy I decided to go through with this surgery. My life and pain levels have improved drastically. I can now go on a walk without worrying if I'll be able to make it home easily. I can kick a soccer ball without residual pain for hours afterward. It has brought me closer to my parents and strengthened my bond with my girlfriend—two things that will stay with me forever, alongside my good and healthy hips. The road to recovery is tough and unpredictable, but that doesn't mean it's a path one shouldn't take.

About Sarah

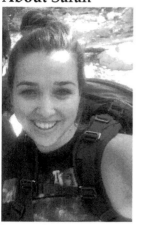

Sarah is 20 years old and a third-year student at the University of California, Santa Cruz, majoring in biology. She has played soccer since she was five and also participated in a club rugby team for her college until she was diagnosed with bilateral acetabular retroversion, very similar to hip dysplasia and entailing the same surgery. She was 18 when she discovered her hips were deformed and only 19 when she underwent her first PAO on December 15, 2014. She has now had her second PAO and first screw removal on June 30, 2015, at age 20, only six months after her first surgery!

Sue Gombis

100 Days

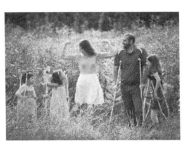

"Make your mess your message."

Have you ever watched the show "Oprah's Master Class"? If not, I highly recommend it. Each episode chronicles the life story of a celebrity, told by the celebrity. But the story is never the pretty, glittery glamour that we often think of when we imagine the life of a celebrity. It's the dirt and grime that helped form them into who they are now. I recently watched an episode about Robin Roberts, who not only fought stereotypes associated with her gender and race to gain respect in the world of sports, but also had to face breast cancer and a blood disorder, fighting just to live. She talked about how fortunate she was to be able to utilize her public status to document her journey as a means of reaching others. She said, "It's knowing you're not alone, it's knowing that somebody else feels the same types of emotions, and trying to learn from each other on how to deal with it." TV is her platform; my blog is mine.

Progress continues to be really slow for me. I have officially spent 100 days on crutches so far this time around. My physical therapist joked a couple weeks ago that it feels like I have spent eight months out of the past year on crutches. When we broke it down, he wasn't too far off. Yikes! My husband doesn't think that 100 days sounds like all that much time (as opposed to saying over three months), but when I sit back and think about it, 100 days sounds like an eternity to me! It was my kids' entire summer vacation, and then some. In that time, we've gone to beaches, water parks and pools, BBQs, bonfires, parties, movies, concerts, and new restaurants; we even managed to make it to Six Flags and go on a boating adventure. Also, J, my daughter, finished her *second* triathlon at the ripe old age of 11! We've done our best to enjoy what we could of the long summer days and warm summer nights. And I did it all on crutches.

My PT just gave me the okay to try going down to one crutch (woo hoo!). I have waited what felt like an eternity to hear him say that. Today, I headed out to the gym for my mini workout (which really only consists of a little biking and a little upper body work) and then planned on running a couple of errands. I left the house with just the one crutch, not wanting to have that second crutch in the car as a backup. Oh, how good it felt to have a free hand again! I'm always a jump-in-feet-first, no-looking-back kind of person when the time comes to ditch crutches. I was 10 minutes into the first errand when the pain became too much on *both* sides, and I had to use a shopping cart as my second crutch. Ugh, I hate being reminded that even this part is a process. And I *hate* having to wonder about the pain on my left side 16 months post op….

I know that my left side complicates recovery for my right side. But I really did go into this surgery thinking my left side would be an afterthought. It's difficult not to compare this recovery to my last, and it's so easy to feel discouraged when things take longer. I think these recoveries depend not only on what we do physically, but also where we are mentally. I have realized the past several weeks that my attitude needed some serious adjusting, and while I'm not always successful at that (there's an understatement), I wonder if I finally got to this point as a result of those efforts. I am hoping that it will only gain momentum from here: maybe using one crutch will boost me emotionally and my more positive attitude will help me to work harder at rehab. Either way, all I can do is continue to try.

I have no idea where this journey will take me. I suppose none of us really do. For a planner and control freak, that's a really scary place to be. I fight the unknown every step of the way: I make plans, I set goals, and I work my tail off to get myself there—so much so, that I feel the disappointment at my core when I fail. I certainly hope the pain on my left side is muscular and will eventually work itself out, but I have to admit that thoughts of arthritis have begun to creep in. There's really no way of knowing at this point. So for now, I'm trying my best to just grab hold as tight as I can, once again, and see where the ride will take me. Roberts said, "To chronicle your own life story is a wonderful gift to give yourself." This is *my* story and I have chosen to share it here until I feel it is finished.

A little taste of my last 100 days:

Celebrating 14 years!
Boating adventures.
First time tubing!
Hold on tight, little man!
Buried in the sand!
Enjoying pool time with my little man!
What's a pool day without a yummy beverage?
Getting ready to tri!!
So crazy proud of this girl, she continues to inspire me to go for what I want, despite how long it takes me.
Special lunch with my girl.
Climbing GIANT trucks...on top of the world, Mom!
Jumping feet first!
First upside-down roller coaster for this guy.
(the little one, not the big one)!
I even managed to get INTO the water....
Enjoying the Chicago Symphony Orchestra...in our own little way.
Yummmmmm.

About Sue

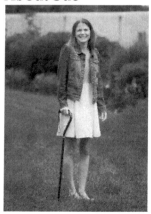

Sue is a mom of three little ones, a wife, an attorney, and a runner/athlete. While training for a half marathon in 2012, she injured her right hip and was diagnosed with FAI and a labral tear. Weeks later, she injured her left hip and was given the same diagnosis. Despite four unsuccessful arthroscopies in less than a year, her first surgeon abandoned her, leaving her to feel like her pain was not real. Sue was devastated. After a couple hours in tears, the fighter in her came out, and she found a hip preservation surgeon who validated her pain and diagnosed her with femoral and acetabular retroversion.

Sue underwent an open dislocation and rotational femoral osteotomy on her left hip in April 2014. Because of the pain caused by the massive hardware, it was removed in October 2014. After a full year of rehab, she was ready for surgery on her right hip, an arthroscopy/PAO in May 2015. When the arthroscopy revealed cartilage damage, her surgeon abandoned the PAO and opted for an open dislocation instead. Sue is now in the thick of rehab, fighting to get my life back for her family and herself.

Chapter 5
Life After Hip Surgery

———— ⌗ ————

"Turn your wounds into wisdom."
Oprah Winfrey

Editor's Note

Life After Hip Surgery

After what may feel like forever, the main phase of PAO recovery will come to an end and one will experience a "new normal." This chapter focuses on the experiences of those who are moving forward after PAO surgery.

In the first narrative, Jessica Dyke contemplates on what life after PAO surgery will hold for her and the best way for her to move forward. Jennifer Sidi reflects on her journey with hip dysplasia, a failed arthroscopic surgery, and two PAO surgeries. She shares her accomplishments and her lessons. Cathy Brett describes the process of which she attained her goal: riding thirty-five miles in the Venus de Miles road (cycling) event. Her success, she explains, has taught her that she is resilient. Jenni Wong portrays her transformative shift through hip dysplasia diagnosis and PAO surgery. Nancy Muir explains her goals of moving past PAO surgery to push herself to run races again. Mary Lynn Bode describes her journey and celebrates her first pain-free day. In the last story, Danielle Gallant shares the letter she wrote to her PAO surgeon one year post-op. Here she eloquently shares her milestones and her lessons.

On a personal note, currently being almost one year post-op on the right hip and 18 months on the left hip, I can say there is life after PAOs. It may not always be easy or pain-free, but I will take my "new normal" any day over my "old normal." As the old saying goes, "That which does kill us makes us stronger."

Jessica Dyke

Crossroads

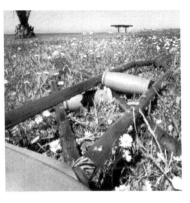

I miss my ski family. I miss Lake Tahoe. I miss the magic of a powder day. I miss shot-skis and hot-tubbing and dance parties in costume. I miss wearing my fart bag. Slicing through the snow, I feel ecstasy in a way I've never been able to find in any other place.

I'm wide-awake at four a.m., feeling raw.

August 21, 2011. Backpacking on the Coast Trail. Wildcat campground. Bass Lake rope swing. Shortly after departing from the swimming spot, my left labrum ripped with one fateful, historic, life-changing step. It was a memorable day. I didn't know it at the time, but my life had just shifted. It's hard to believe it's been over four years since my hip dysplasia saga began. Too many years. I can't think about that, though.

August 21, 2011, is also the last time I saw my friend Seth. A week later, he was killed by a falling tree. We would daydream together sometimes. We would plot how we'd quit our jobs and move to a ski town. That's when I threw myself into my Great Escape plans—hip pain be damned. *I'm alive,* I thought. It's time to truly live. He died, and it changed me. I wouldn't follow the big dreams just for me. I'd do it for both of us.

I wish I knew what it all means. I wish I had some profound revelation, some pretty words to pack it up in. But I don't.

I do know that I am approaching a crossroads. What comes after PAOs? The thought of going back to the job that has siphoned the life force out of me makes me nauseous. Returning to the status quo is simply not acceptable. I'm obviously beyond desperate for change, but I'm afraid. I fear that I won't have the courage to break free. I fear that my body won't be able to do all the things I dream of doing. I fear that I won't have the guts to grab life by the balls.

Maybe what it all means is that life is too precious to spend paralyzed by fear. We must keep moving forward, even if moving forward sometimes means sitting still. The PAO life has forced me to slow down and experience what it means to truly face oneself. It hasn't always been comfortable, but the growth is worth it. Soon it will be time to chart new territory. I must follow my heart, take risks, and accept that there are no guarantees in life. They say that the only way out is through. When I reach the crossroads, I know what I need to do. I will step into the flames and face my fears. I will trust that this path is full of treasures beyond my wyldest dreams.

About Jessica

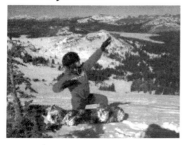

The Juicer is a warrior. She is a seeker of adventure, depth, and truth. She stares intently into the abyss, dreaming of intriguing possibilities. She will boldly step into the flames and let the fire burn away the debris. She is tectonically shifting into a life beyond her wyldest fantasies.

Her hip saga began on August 21, 2011, when she tore her labrum while backpacking on the northern California coast. Since then, she has had two PAOs by two different surgeons in 2013 and 2014, one screw-removal surgery in 2015, and will most likely undergo a follow-up surgery in 2016 to fix a rare complication—unattached abdominal muscles—as a result of her LPAO.

She is a master at seizing every magnificent moment of life and is currently on a journey of self-awareness and discovery. She's beating her wings yet, knowing that someday soon she will be the Phoenix rising from the ashes of all her fears and setbacks.

Want to ride the Juicer train? Best have courage of mind, body, and spirit. Throw off your armor and open your heart. Destination—SOULSDEEP.

You may follow her journey through PAO life at juiceyblogsack.wordpress.com.

Jennifer Sidi

PAO Hip Story

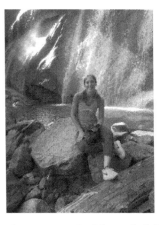

It's not about wanting to go under the knife; it's about wanting to be "fixed." I started to lose hope that would ever happen. You come to learn that in order to be "fixed," you have to find the root of the problem. Although that may sound simple, it took more than five years and three failed surgeries for that to happen to me.

I thought the problem was my knees, so I saw a knee orthopedist. Then, I thought it was my back, so I saw a spinal specialist. I went through years of physical therapy, and although I lived my life, it was not to the extent that I wanted to. It finally took a physical therapist to tell me it may be my hips, when I complained of that infamous groin pain.

I wish I could say the story ended there. I wish I could say I found the hip specialist, had surgery, and was completely better. I guess I should have been suspicious. The original hip surgeon told me my hips were not normal on the X-ray and that I would likely need early hip replacements. I did not even care. I just wanted to be out of pain and back to the life a woman in her twenties should be living. It took two MRIs to find the torn labrum. The surgery was promised to be easy, and it was! I was out of work as a labor and delivery nurse for less than two weeks. I went home with a cane and did not even need it the next day. The pain was minimal, and I immediately felt better. If only it lasted…

Well, it did last, kind of. For about eighteen months I was pain free, but while driving home from a friend who lived 120 miles away from me, that pain came back. It was intense, and I'm not sure which was more painful: the actual pain or that fact that I knew something was wrong again.

I saw my surgeon, and the MRI did not show a new tear, although I was almost hoping it would. I wanted an explanation! I think so many of us understand that feeling. However, my surgeon was on my side! He knew something was wrong and wanted to go back in with the scope again and look in the joint. The surgery was long, and I woke up in recovery about six or seven hours after initially heading into the operating room. I clearly remember the physician's fellow telling me the cartilage was in very bad shape and I would likely need a hip replacement within five to 10 years. It was a little hard to comprehend after just waking up from general anesthesia, but when I could think clearly, I realized it meant I would likely be getting a new hip before I even turned 35.

The recovery was longer this time, as there was some shaving of the bone, and I was on crutches for about four weeks. At my six-week post-operative appointment, I went back to the surgeon in tears. The pain was back, and my heart knew it was not post-operative pain. My hip gave out on me right before the appointment. I actually fell trying to get into the house because the hip just slipped. I figured the surgeon would tell me I needed to give healing more time, and he did mention that he really thought I would need the replacement sooner than later. By my three-month post-op appointment, he was certain of that.

As any responsible patient, I wanted to get another opinion at this point. I was upset and overwhelmed. I also had built up my career in my hospital and was scared stiff to tell my very kind manager that I may need another surgery when I literally had just gotten back to work. Fast-forward to one more failed hip surgery to create a graft for my trashed capsule, and then I re-discovered a surgeon who gave me the option for the scariest surgery, but one that might actually do the trick and save my hip from a replacement at such a young age. I say the word "re-discover" because I had met him after surgery number two but was steered in another direction, which is where the capsule reconstruction came into play. It was also discovered after hip surgery #3 that the labrum on the other hip was torn and frayed, and I knew in my heart that hip may be looking at the same fate.

The PAO, as we all know, is no joke. It's a major surgery with possibly severe complications. However, the possibility of complications didn't faze me because I was tired! Tired of pain, tired of failed surgeries, and tired of not being able to be active. I was tired of having issues at work and tired of people questioning about all the surgeries and why they didn't work. I didn't know why they didn't work until a brilliant surgeon with an awesome bedside manner explained it to me.

March 26, 2014, and April 8, 2015, are dates that I will never forget. I can honestly tell you I do not remember the dates of any of the other three surgeries. However, PAO number one and PAO number two have become permanently ingrained into my mind. Those two days were not easy by any means, but they became life-changers. They became the days that I know a surgeon worked damn hard to give me back what I wanted and needed. He worked hard to ensure that I could have quality of life and longevity of my hip joints. Those two days are the reason that I was able to complete an intense hike up to waterfalls that would not have been seen otherwise. They are the reason I was able to keep up with an Ironman twin sister in rock climbing and training. I may never have perfect hips, but I now have very functional ones. I feel strong and ready to take on more than I ever thought my body was capable of.

Hip dysplasia may have given me hardship, but it also taught me more about life than I thought possible. I am able to embrace the hardship, to turn it into strength for my lifetime. Hip dysplasia even allowed me to create bonds with people I never knew beforehand. Every life experience opens up opportunity for growth and learning, and that even includes the ones that cause us extreme hardship. My life would have been easier without five hip surgeries; however, it has 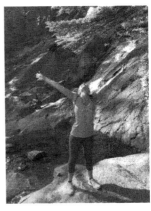 become richer because of what I have been through. It taught me lessons that I can now instill in my own patients whom I care for. It allowed me to realize I had strength I never knew existed. For those of you who have had the surgery: I know those early days are tough, but remember, there is always a finish line somewhere. I don't know for sure that I have reached it, but it is coming closer, and I now have strong motivation to cross it.

About Jennifer

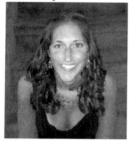

Jennifer Sidi is a 32-year-old from Long Island, New York. She has been working as a registered nurse for more than 10 years, with the past eight years in the labor and delivery unit of a busy hospital on Long Island. She is currently pursuing a nurse practitioner degree. In her limited spare time, she enjoys traveling, skating, the beach, Netflix (for downtime), and the gym. At this time she thoroughly enjoys putting her corrected hips to the test with any new and challenging activity!

Cathy Brett

20-Degree Shift—A New Angle of Resilient

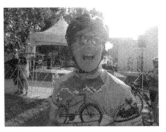

I have been blessed with a physical body that has always been strong, coordinated, stable, healthy, balanced, and able to endure crazy adventures and hold up longer than I thought I could...until I didn't.

We all have moments in life when we are forced to pause, to stop our world and re-evaluate. I sat in my car for a long time after seeing the hip specialist who broke the news to me that not only did I have "full blown" bilateral hip dysplasia, but also as a bonus, my right labrum was shredded. My center-edge (CE) angle measured approximately 10 degrees. Go figure, congenital dysplasia and just now finding out at age 49. I had played collegiate volleyball and completed a marathon, half marathons, week-long bike rides, triathlons, backpacking, hiking, rock climbing, back-flips on the trampoline, and had no idea. That was a big pause for me.

Luckily, still being a candidate for PAO, I opted to have the surgeries. In a two-month period, I had labrum reconstruction and my femoral head was reshaped followed by a right PAO, resulting in a much-improved CE angle by rotating the acetabulum 20 degrees.

My doctors were very upfront about the complexity and the long healing process, especially with me being older. I didn't quite appreciate the complexity until I was in the thick of it. This has absolutely been one of the hardest things I have been through, with limited activity, dependency on others for even the simplest of daily tasks, and mentally sitting with my hurting self day in, day out. On those hardest days, I leaned on my friends and family, I leaned on the PAO groups, and I leaned on myself to find out how resilient I am.

It has been a long year getting re-acquainted with my glutes and all the other muscles, nerves, and bones that were part of the 20-degree shift. My disruptive twenty-degree shift has given me the opportunity to celebrate, to love and honor my body for what it can do each day, and to simply embrace the little things.

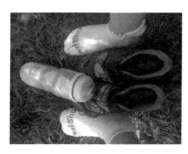

I am a road cyclist. It is my outlet, it is my mental escape, and it is my way of seeing beautiful places and sharing fun memories with friends. It took nearly eight months before my body was cooperating enough to clip into my pedals and get back in the saddle. During the first several weeks, I had to honor the fact that I was at a place were I could be more of a deterrent than a benefit to myself. My limit was to ride no more than five miles. Although feeling a little bit silly putting on lycra and my jersey to ride five miles, I still did it. I got up early before work this summer and road five miles a few times a week. Then, I went to six miles and each week, increased the frequency and the mileage by one or two miles. I had a goal to ride in an organized ride with several of my amazing friends who were my caretakers. As the ride approached and I did the math, I didn't have enough time to just add one mile each week. The ride I signed up for was 30 miles. So, with the blessing of my PT, I started pushing double-digit mileage rides: 10, 12, 14 and 21 miles. Each time I went further pushing new limits, it gave me yet another moment to pause and get familiar with my body within my 20-degree angle shift.

And happily, on August 29, 2015, I rode my bike 34 miles in the Venus de Miles. There were tears of joy and relief as I celebrated with the amazing friends who have stood by me, cared for me, drove me, dressed me, made sure I took my meds, and loved me. They each have told me how resilient I am. And I've learned from this new 20-degree angle shift that I am resilient. This PAO journey has given me better days and forever shifted me and those around me.

About Cathy

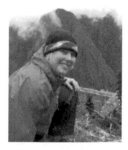

Cathy Brett is a 51-year-old, gypsy-spirited and life-long adventurer living in Fort Collins, Colorado. Since her surgery, she embraces each step she is able to take with tremendous gratitude, knowing each day is truly a gift.

Jenni Wong

Shy Gal to Cheerleader

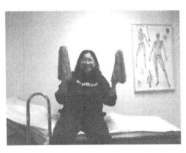

Hip dysplasia is real. It has forever changed my life, rocking my world in all directions imaginable, changing me physically and emotionally. The experiences and challenges I've overcome have tempered my soul and renewed my love for life. It's unbelievable how much a person's persona can change after diagnosis and treatment of bilateral hip dysplasia. Ultimately, I had to have a major hip surgery called periacetabular osteotomy (PAO), the process that transformed me from a shy, introverted gal into a vocal and gregarious warrior. As bizarre as it may sound, I'm utterly grateful to be on this PAO journey. The massive amount of medical research, decision making, and support needed to survive this process are the key things that forced me out of my comfortable shell and turned me into a PAO Warrior Cheerleader for a group of amazing and courageous individuals.

For 38 years, I was a quiet and reserved person. It was daunting for me to speak honestly with people held in high regard in society, like medical professionals. Everything changed in October 2013 when I started experiencing groin and hip pain after workouts. I thought I pulled a muscle; boy, was I wrong! I didn't really know what to make of the pain, so for four months I just tried to limit my workouts and leisurely exercised in hopes it would go away. My pain kept getting worse, so at my annual physical in January 2014, just two months shy of turning the BIG 40, I decided to be honest about my sore hips with my doctor. Unbeknownst to me, my quiet universe was about to be transformed into a big ball of crazy.

February to December 2014 was filled with medical uncertainty, referrals to the wrong doctors, insurance issues, multiple tests, appointments, and two months of unsuccessful physical therapy in an attempt to relieve soreness. I was beyond confused, frustrated, and I seriously considered giving up and living with hip pain. That's when I started to get angry, and that anger fueled a fire inside me that I never knew existed. I learned to advocate for my medical needs. Advocating for my health led to a meeting in July 2014 with an orthopedic surgeon by the name of Dr. Michael Bellino who specializes in PAOs at Stanford Hospital. On December 9, 2014, he performed a PAO on my right hip.

The six nights, seven days in the hospital were tough: the rapid response team was called twice, once for respiratory distress due to medications and again for a seizure-like episode, which was later diagnosed by a neurologist to be a physical response due to anxiety, metabolic imbalances, and low red blood cell count. I recovered after some blood transfusions and was able to start recovery at home, which also wasn't exactly a walk in the park. But as hard as it's been, I'm grateful I was able to have this surgery and will forever be thankful to Dr. Bellino. He's an amazing surgeon who genuinely cares about his patients and was instrumental in guiding me to the wonderful periacetabular osteotomy (PAO) support group on Facebook. I never would've survived my PAO without this support network, nor would I have become a PAO Cheerleader if my friend, mentor, and fellow PAO Warrior, Jen Lesea-Ames, hadn't bestowed the role upon me.

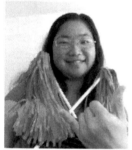

Throughout my PAO journey, I've learned how to engage with people better and be more vocal; it's been a true education in connecting with people. The encouragement from the support group inspired me to pay it forward by supporting others. My cheerleading role in the group became official during a PAO lunch meet-up with Jen and other warriors. There she presented me with a set of green mini pom-poms and dubbed me the PAO Cheerleader of the group for the positive support I'd given. Everyone at the table let me to know they were there to support me as well, since they knew I have also been a little overwhelmed with trying to support my mother with her struggles of dealing with peritoneal kidney dialysis at home. The generous remarks and kind gift caught me off guard: shy, quiet me, the cheerleader? I was shocked yet honored at the same time, what an overwhelming joyful moment in my life! After the luncheon, I posted a thank-you to Jen on our support group's Facebook page, and she posted back with a friendly dare: take the pom-poms to my post-op appointment with Dr. Bellino the following week and give him a CHEER! I hoped she was joking, but she and the other warriors in the support group continued to enthusiastically encourage me to do the cheer. The thought terrified me, but I started thinking about just how far I'd come since joining the support group, and I knew Jen had suggested the dare to help me get over my nervousness at doctor appointments. She felt I could get over my nerves if I could just maybe get my doctor to laugh and share some smiles.

My appointment day came up quickly, and I hesitantly stuck the pom-poms in my backpack as I headed to Stanford. When I got there I did my X-rays and nervously sat in the waiting room while pondering my dare. My name was called; it was now or never! I sat on the examination table staring at my backpack knowing the dreaded pom-poms were in there. I knew that if I didn't take them out and place them by me, I might totally chicken out. I bravely got off the examination table, took the pom-poms out, and placed them at the end of the table. My heart wanted to pop out of my chest, and I was sweating bullets. Before I had the chance to chicken out, there was a knock at the door and in walked Dr. Bellino. He smiled when he saw the fluorescent green pom-poms, remarking that he couldn't wait to hear the story behind those after we finished the exam. This light interaction had already made me more comfortable; maybe Jen was on to something!

The appointment was almost over when he brought up the pom-poms, as he was curious to know the story. I shared with him how Jen had given me the pom-poms, the PAO Cheerleader backstory, and the dare to give him a cheer. To my utter shock, he rolled back in his chair and said with a big grin, "So, am I going to get a CHEER?" Cue stage fright. I didn't know why I was so nervous because, after all, I do trust this wonderful surgeon. He'd helped me so much, and I feel much better than before surgery, so he deserved this. So as nervous as I was, I put on my best smile, grabbed the pom-poms, and prepared to give my cheer. Just as I was about to raise the pom-poms up into the air, he stopped me. "Oh, wait! We need proof or how will Jen know you did it? Let's take a video of it!"

At this point my anxiety was getting the best of me, and I couldn't think straight, so I squeaked, "NO, IT'S OK! We don't need a video, plus I don't have my phone handy." He brushed that right off and proceeded to grab his phone from his pocket. Oh no, no, no... The nerves are coming on stronger, and shy me was back! I couldn't believe I was doing this at all. In an effort to stall, I said, "OH WAIT! My phone's there in the mesh pocket of my backpack!" I grabbed it and handed it to him. There's no chickening out now! He leaned back in his roller chair and was about to take the photo, but then paused again. My heart dropped as my anxiety went through the roof. He smiled and just asked me to scoot closer to the skeleton poster to make it obvious the picture was taken in his office. Then it was time.

I simply shouted, "YAHOO!!! I'm feeling GREAT!" as he snapped the picture. That was all I felt that I needed to say, that one cheer encapsulating my joy in having my hip fixed, life changed, and friends made forever.

I felt surreal afterwards because my intense shyness wouldn't have let me do that in the past, and I told Dr. Bellino. He responded with, "It's OK Jenni, I'm really shy, too, so that makes two of us." His reply solidified for me why I'm so blessed to have him as my surgeon. He not only fixed my hip but helped turn a once shy gal into an outgoing PAO Warrior who loves to support others in our PAO community. I'm whole-heartedly thankful for all the people I've connected with and for all the support. As I continue on my PAO journey, I will be using this incredible experience as a tool to continue to be the best PAO Cheerleader for all PAO Warriors in the amazing Facebook PAO support group.

About Jenni

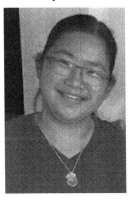

Aloha! Jenni Wong is a 41-year-old PAO Warrior. She was born and raised in San Jose, California, and is proud of her Hawaiian style upbringing. Her parents are originally from Oahu, Hawaii, and although they chose to raise her and her twin sister on the mainland, they raised them with what island folks like to call "The Aloha Spirit." The Aloha Spirit in essence means to treat everyone like ohana ("family" in Hawaiian): to be friendly, loving, and compassionate, and to help others whenever and wherever possible.

Jenni prides herself in having this spirit of Aloha, so as shy and introverted as she may be, she strives to do her best to spread the Aloha Spirit to others, whether it's in her personal life, in her profession as a youth and teen recreation coordinator, in her new-found love of visiting fellow PAO Warriors in the hospital, and in supporting fellow warriors via their Facebook group page. She's forever grateful for this PAO surgery because it has truly changed her, making her a better human being. Mahalo!

Nancy Muir

Story of a Future Data Point

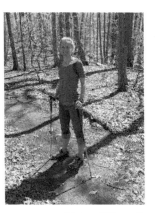

A possible stress fracture? That would be the worst thing ever! (Should I mention I can be dramatic?)

The deep, dull ache set in around mile 17 of my 24th marathon. When it didn't go away, I responded like many other distance runners—I promptly ignored the pain and ran a 50-kilometer race the next weekend.

When the pain still didn't go away, I grudgingly decided to go visit the free runner's injury clinic. I was expecting the sports medicine PT to diagnose me with bursitis or tendinitis; instead, she agreed that my symptoms didn't seem consistent with any of the more traditional running injuries. Her strong opinion was the following: don't run again until getting an X-ray to rule out a stress fracture.

So, instead of running a local 50-kilometer race two days later, I found myself staring at X-rays in an orthopedic surgeon's office. And instead of hearing words like "stress fracture" and "no running for six to eight weeks," I was introduced to words such as "Ganz," "osteotomy," "dysplasia," "total hip replacement," "joint deterioration," and "major activity modifications."

One of the greatest ironies is that hip dysplasia was not a new concept to me. As a pediatric physical therapist, I regularly screen all young infants I evaluate for hip dysplasia. I educate parents of children with developmental, neurological, and musculoskeletal conditions on positioning to optimize hip development, and I have spent countless weekend hours calling around to local stores trying to track down car seats that will accommodate a spica cast in order to safely discharge young patients home from the hospital after hip surgery.

Hip dysplasia in my pediatric patients, yes. But hip dysplasia in a 31-year-old who had logged more than 30,000 running miles on her hips over the course of 17 years without even developing so much as shin splints or knee pain? No.

By the time I met with a surgeon who had experience in PAOs, I had read every article I could find about adult hip dysplasia and PAOs. I knew the history of the procedure, the reported long-term outcomes, alternatives to osteotomy procedures, prognostic factors, and even the intrarater reliability of the radiological angle measurements.

I still didn't believe that any of this actually had to do with me. Over the next several months, I talked to 10 different surgeons, including hip preservation specialists, hip replacement specialists, and surgeons who specialize in arthroscopy. Although it was not what I wanted to hear, there was reassurance that came with the mutual consensus: yes, I had hip dysplasia; yes, the internal damage I already caused to my labrum and cartilage was "not insignificant"; and, yes, I was an excellent candidate for a PAO. What was less reassuring was that all of the surgeons agreed that my current level of function was higher than most patients who decide to pursue a PAO, that no one could predict how quickly my joint status might progress to the point that I would no longer be a good surgery candidate, and that no one could guarantee that I would get back to my current level of function after surgery—or whether trying would be advisable.

For me, the PAO and immediate recovery were the easy parts. I had an incredible support system, no complications, and minimal pain. My overall rehabilitation has been relatively quick and seamless. Overall, my current function is high: I can hike for hours; have taken up mountain biking; am able to effortlessly and painlessly care for my home and my yard; and I'm able to squat, jump, crawl, and climb to keep up with my young patients all day at work.

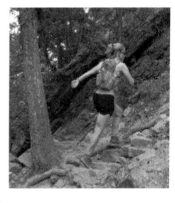

However, the challenges, frustrations, and fears continue.

The body that I always trusted suddenly seems foreign; I no longer know which way my feet should turn when I walk, squat, and jump, and the once-therapeutic motion of running reduces me to a limp within seconds. I find myself struggling with intermittent back pain, knee pain, and sacroiliac pain that I've never had before, and given that I had minimal joint pain pre- or post-operatively, I don't trust myself to distinguish good pain from potentially damaging pain. While my symptoms remain minimal, my other hip is borderline dysplastic and both knees have dysplastic features; I stress over every twinge of discomfort. My PT and surgeon don't seem to know what to say regarding pain or outcome except that I'm still early in the recovery process and that I need to give it at least a year. Maybe two.

My surgeon told me once that he knew that patience with the recovery process was going to be a far greater challenge for me than the actual PAO. There is definite truth in this. It is, however, a great challenge to be a statistical data point that has yet to be analyzed. The research on PAOs has historically defined success of this procedure on "survivorship" of the joint or, in other words, joints that don't need to be converted to total hip replacements during the study period. More recently, a few studies have started to look at more functional and quality-of-life outcomes: what are patients able to do post-operatively and how satisfied are they with the outcomes? The anecdotes I hear from other physically active patients following PAO are inspiring and motivating, but there is no literature that looks specifically at long-term survivorship of these hips.

So what do I do with this?

I have learned enough to know that even the aggressive PAO surgery does not restore normal hip mechanics and is not performed with the goal of restoring high levels of physical function. The PT and rationalizer in me starts thinking about ground reaction forces, shallow acetabula, early degenerative changes, the anchors in my labrum, and the stitches in my joint capsule and confesses that, perhaps, long-term repetitive pounding, quick direction changes, and guaranteed face plants on the trails may be a bit ironic following "joint preservation" surgery. I think about the potential implications of future joint pain and deformity on my personal, professional, mental, and financial futures and grapple with what my long-term life priorities may look like. My life is good. The surgery went well, and there are many activities that I can enjoy without pain. Should I stop while I'm ahead?

But the runner and researcher in me still wants to continue to test my limits. Those parts of me still want to see just how far I can push myself physically, mentally, and emotionally. Can I complete another 50-miler? Or a 100-miler? Or maybe longer? The runner in me misses those quiet, foggy mornings on the trail, nighttime runs with just the illumination of a headlamp in the dark woods, the intimate conversations that happen only on the trails between otherwise unlikely friends, the excitement of conquering a new distance or a new time, the smell of new running shoes, dirt on the car mats, and the exhilaration that comes from being awarded with a spectacular view at the top of a steep climb. And I'm not sure I'm ready to give that all up quite yet.

And maybe, by pushing the limits, I can aspire to more data points.

About Nancy

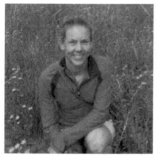

Nancy is a 33-year-old pediatric physical therapist who lives and works in Cincinnati, Ohio. When she's not busy driving her PT crazy or trying to keep up with the amazing kids who inspire and challenge (and positively exhaust!) her at work on a daily basis, you can find her with her trekking poles or mountain bike "navigating" (a.k.a. frequently getting lost in) the trail systems across Cincinnati and northern Kentucky, snuggling with her special-needs kitties, eating, traveling, delving into her post-graduate studies, developing IRB proposals to learn more about rehabilitation and functional outcomes after PAO surgery, and dreaming of her next big trail ultra-running adventure. Nancy continues to be terrified of blisters and stress fractures.

Mary Lynn Bode

My Journey Through Hip Dysplasia

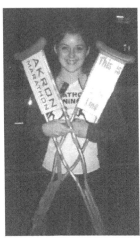

I was completely submerged, feeling the pressure on my lungs as I sunk further and further. All the sounds around me blended together into one droning mumble as I gasped for air. The colors glistened as the images around me were smudged into nothingness. The pressure on my chest became too much to bear; I couldn't breathe. Flickers of light passed my eyes as I could feel the top layer of the water. Sucking in the only oxygen available, my nostrils were barely above the waterline. I've lost control, I don't know how I got here, and I don't know how to get out. I was lost and submerged in questions about why I was in so much pain, why I was told again and again, "There's nothing wrong."

I was 12 years old when the most severe pain started in my hip. I woke up one day and couldn't put any weight on my leg. I was told my X-ray looked normal and was sent on my way with crutches and no answers. I couldn't walk, play with my friends, or even sleep through the night without waking up with severe pain. However, I was told nothing was wrong. So, I started to convince myself that this was true.

I was on the cross-country team and was told that pain was normal when you ran. "No pain, no gain" was the term used. I slowly started to believe it and chose to stop fighting the pain and learned to deal with it. Years went by, and the pain started to get worse, and worse, and worse. However, I was still in denial. I started to train for a marathon. Yes, a full 26.2-mile marathon. I was in the prime time in my life. I had just graduated college and got a job right away. Finishing a full marathon was my dream. As I trained, I envisioned myself running through the finish line after hours of sweat and exhaustion. I yearned for that feeling of accomplishment, exhilaration, and determination, knowing I spent months training for this very moment.

However, my hip had other plans. My dream was ripped away from me halfway through training. While I was on my 16-mile run, I got a stress fracture in my hip. I was told immediately to go on crutches, while I was sent from surgeon to surgeon. I had diagnoses from cancer to a shrug of the shoulders. No one knew why a 20-year-old female had a stress fracture, large ganglion cysts, and a torn labrum. During this time, I was forced to quit my job and started going back to school—something I could do sitting down most of the day. Finally, after three months, a team of surgeons got together to look at my case. I was then sent to Dr. W., a surgeon who specialized in a surgery called periacetabular osteotomy.

Dr. W. looked at my X-ray, turned around instantly, looked me in the eyes, and said, "You have hip dysplasia, there's no doubt about that." There was that feeling again, that pressure on my chest, feeling like I could barely hold on, the water filling up. My heart felt like it dropped into my stomach. His explanation of what to expect next blended together as I strained to hold back the tears. "Stay strong; it's going to be OK." I just kept repeating these words to myself. As my sister and mother sat listening to the surgeons explanation of how my life was going to change forever, my mind blurred. My entire life changed in that moment, as I embarked on a life-changing surgery.

As I was finishing the school year, I scheduled my surgery five months later. Those were some of the most difficult five months of my life. The pain—so much pain—but I was still in denial. I was told again and again from people that met me, "You're too young to have a cane." But what was even more piercing were the judgmental stares from random strangers. I imagined what they were thinking, "Why does she have that cane?" "What's wrong with her?" "Is she faking it?" The feelings of embarrassment were too overwhelming. So, one day I left my cane in the car and went to class that was two buildings away from the parking lot. This was the day I would come to accept that I had hip dysplasia. I walked out of the classroom, after class had finished, and started walking back to my car. I only made it 100 feet when I couldn't put any weight on my leg. The knife-like pain was so intense, I couldn't think straight. I needed my cane. This very distinct moment replays in my mind to this day. The stark white hallway, no chairs anywhere to be seen, the bright searing lights, people passing by with those judgmental stares, that feeling again. Water rushing in, I couldn't breathe. No one asked if I was okay; no one came to help. I was on my own in the middle of nowhere, stranded. I needed help, I needed my cane, and right then I knew I needed this surgery.

Finally, it was surgery day, PAO Warrior Day. I woke up with that feeling: submerged in questions, anxiety, what-ifs. The water level was at its peak. No oxygen left, just residual leftover from the months of worry. My thoughts consumed me as I was left alone in a hospital room waiting for them to prep me for surgery. My thoughts raced around in my head. The only thing that got me through was the thought that maybe, just maybe, I could actually have a day, a moment, where I wasn't in pain. This was the only way that was going to happen. This surgery was my only chance.

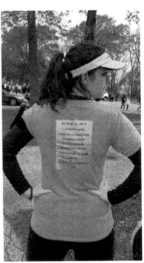

After nine months of intense recovery after my PAO, I finally had that day without pain! I continued to start having weeks without pain, then months. I was able to become a normal person again, do normal things, and not think about my hip every moment of every day. No longer did the water rush in from worry, I could breathe again, live again, RUN AGAIN! I proudly tell my story because it is a success story. I am a PAO Warrior, and I have Persevered And Overcome the pain of hip dysplasia. Take *that*, hip dysplasia!

About Mary Lynn

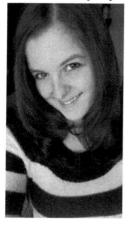

Mary Lynn Bode is an occupational therapy master's student at Cleveland State University. She found a love for healthcare and helping others through her own medical challenges that started early in life. She is incredibly fortunate to have an unbelievable support system that helped her through this entire hip dysplasia journey. Her family and friends supported her through every moment and were the reason why she had such success in recovery. From visiting her in the hospital, to sitting with her all day, to bringing entertaining occupations to pass the time, to pushing her through stores in a wheelchair, to just holding her hand when the pain was too much to bear, her family and friends were her rock.

Mary Lynn enjoys spending time with friends and family, yoga, running, swimming, photography, brewing beer, and taking hikes in the park with her fiancé, Chris.

She was diagnosed with hip dysplasia when she was 21 years old after training for a full marathon. Shortly after, she had an LPAO on May 14, 2012.

"Anyone can give up, it's the easiest thing in the world to do.
But to hold it together when everyone else would
understand if you fell apart, that's true strength."
Unknown

Danielle Gallant

Gratitude, Abound: A Letter to My Surgeon on My One-Year PAO-a-versary

To my most favorite doctor,

I need you to know my life is totally different now.

I've spent a lot of time thinking about how I could write this letter to you, and many times I've seemed to come up short, not able to relay my true level of gratefulness. I've found it to be impossible to fully put into words. However, I'm going to try.

Before PAO, my life was based on decisions—decisions that were completely dictated by levels of pain. "Can I go to the store after work? Or will my hip hurt too much by then?" "It's Saturday, but we can only run two errands because I can't walk for more than a few minutes at a time." "I should take a carriage around the grocery store, I will need it to help me get around." "How many pain killers should I take this morning to dull the pain?"

Many days I was too exhausted to even think about running errands. My hip had gotten best of me more often than I care to admit.

I have to be honest: I had lived with it for so long that I really didn't even know how bad it really was. It was just life as I knew it. I didn't know how bad it was until I was good. I am now so good.

As I progress in my recovery, it is becoming clearer and clearer how much this surgery has genuinely changed my life. It was life changing. Those words are often used in a dramatic fashion but in this instance they are completely 100% true.

My milestones have been plentiful and happen rather often. I don't want to bore you with what seems like the millions of amazing moments since my PAO surgery, but I do feel like I need to share some of these things with you. You need to understand just how meaningful your work is and how much life you have given back to me.

My youngest brother got married in June. I was ecstatic two years ago when I was chosen as a bridesmaid, and I knew I'd be pretty far along in recovery by then. His wedding became one of my personal major milestones for recovery. I knew that not only did I want to walk down the aisle with no assistance devices, but I also wanted to walk down the aisle pain-free. On June 15, I completed my task as bridesmaid. Better yet, I reached my personal goal and walked down the aisle at my brother's wedding. Instead of limping down the aisle and worrying about my hip buckling in pain, I watched my brother's face glow as he prepared to see his bride. That was a really fantastic moment for me personally and was an emotional moment for my family.

In August, Matt (my husband) and I traveled to California. We spent eight days seeing the sites and taking in as much of San Francisco and Los Angeles as we could. Leading up to vacation, I had worked hard at physical therapy to get to a point where I could walk correctly, pain-free, and without fatigue for the entire trip. I am happy to tell you that not only did I not have any pain at all in the hip throughout the entire trip, but also there were also two different days that I logged over 10,000 steps. One of these days, I walked 18,000 steps. 18,000 steps! An entire day of walking the hills of San Francisco, and I didn't need to stop once to rest because my hip hurt too much. And while that is an amazing feat in and of itself, what is even more amazing is that I didn't even think of my hip that day. Dr. Schiller, I walked 18,000 steps without even thinking about my hip. At the end of the day, I glanced down at my pedometer and nearly cried with joy. That may seem silly, but that is something I've never experienced.

These events, with the tens of thousands of steps, are now frequent from week to week. I am doing things every day that I never ever would have even thought of doing. I am doing 12- to 14-hour workdays in the woods, and I'm not even batting an eye. I can walk, hike, climb, step…I can do everything that I should have always been able to do.

This recovery has taught me many, many things. It's taught me patience and more patience (and then more patience). It's taught me how to ask for help when I need it and to accept it when it's offered. It's taught me that it's okay to rely on others; if you surround yourself with the right people, they'll always come through. It's taught me the meaning of hard work, and that physical therapy is not just physical…it's mental therapy, too.

This recovery has taught me many, many things. However, of all the things I've learned, the most important thing I've learned is gratitude. I wake up every day and the first thing I think of is how grateful I am for my new hip. Every time I get up from my chair, or I stroll across the parking lot at work, or I even just get up to go to the kitchen in my house, I am grateful. I am grateful for comfortable sitting positions and to sleep soundly through the night. I am thankful for long days out and about with my husband, Matt. I am thankful for never having to turn down a day of shopping with my mom because my hip will never be able to keep up. I am grateful for a normal life, doing normal things. I am so filled with gratitude that I am bursting at the seams.

Above every other thing, I am most thankful for you. I am thankful that I found University Orthopedics and that I somehow made my way into your care. I am thankful for your talents, for your support, and for your encouragement. What you've given me is worth more than any amount of money in the world. Thank you for every single appointment, for the diagnosis, and for the recommendation of PAO. Thank you for completing the surgery in such a skillful way so that I can be where I am today. I've been blessed to have such a seamless recovery from such a daunting procedure... that is all, no doubt, because of you. So, thank you. I am forever grateful for this new life that I am living. I will be sure to never, ever take a moment of it for granted.

About Danielle

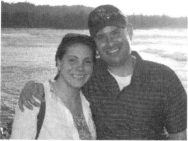

Danielle is 30 years old and from New England in the United States. She is an environmental scientist, and she loves to spend her days walking through the woods, watching birds, taking pictures, baking, and sipping coffee. She is married to a wonderful man and has a wonderful family who have given nothing but unwavering support throughout her hip journey.

Danielle was born with developmental dysplasia of the hips (DDH), and her surgical hip journey began in 2010 when she learned that she needed a right periacetabular osteotomy (RPAO) to correct this. She had RPAO in 2012, followed by right arthroscopic surgery in 2013 to repair labral damage. While her recovery was long and hard, the surgeries were wildly successful, and she is living every day pain-free! Danielle would like to thank all of her friends and family who helped her recover smoothly from such a daunting procedure. She feels she truly could not have done it without your love and support! Between the meal donations, the help with house cleaning, the constant company... she can never fully express her gratitude and feels so lucky.

Chapter Six
Poems

"A happy life consists not in the absence,
but in the mastery of hardships."
Helen Keller

Editor's Note

Poems

Sometimes poems express the experience better than a narrative essay. In this last chapter, we have a collection of poems.

Jenni Wong gives meaning to "Our Challenge," while Wendy Thomas gives meaning to "Periacetabular Osteotomy, Hip Dysplasia." Laura Ricci's poem describes her wish to have a better functioning, pain-free hip. Jill Campbell's Haiku describes the PAO surgery and recovery. The last poem, "Ode to a Hip," was written by Geraldine O'Sullivan, roommate to a PAO Warrior.

The poems encompass all aspects of this journey. I hope you enjoy reading them.

Jenni Wong

The PAO—Our CHALLENGE

Courageous and tenacious survivors

Hip warriors

Actively working towards their goals

Living their lives to the fullest

Lending support to their fellow PAO Warriors

Enduring every emotion imaginable

Never giving up

Grateful to their surgeon

Excelling and persevering everyday

About Jenni

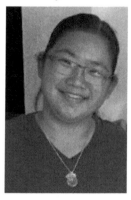

Aloha! Jenni Wong is a 41-year-old PAO Warrior. She was born and raised in San Jose, California, and is proud of her Hawaiian style upbringing. Her parents are originally from Oahu, Hawaii, and although they chose to raise her and her twin sister on the mainland, they raised them with what island folks like to call "The Aloha Spirit." The Aloha Spirit in essence means to treat everyone like ohana ("family" in Hawaiian): to be friendly, loving, and compassionate, and to help others whenever and wherever possible.

Jenni prides herself in having this spirit of Aloha, so as shy and introverted as she may be, she strives to do her best to spread the Aloha Spirit to others, whether it's in her personal life, in her profession as a youth and teen recreation coordinator, in her new-found love of visiting fellow PAO Warriors in the hospital, and in supporting fellow warriors via their Facebook group page. She's forever grateful for this PAO surgery because it has truly changed her, making her a better human being. Mahalo!

Wendy Thomas

PERIACETABULAR OSTEOTOMY, HIP DYSPLASIA

Pain

Enduring

Rigor

Independence

Agony

Consultants

Elasticated stockings

Tinzaparin injections

All together

Battle

United

Love between warriors

Anger

Relatives

Old

Strength

Tension

Exercises

Overbearing

Tormented

Outlook

Medication

Young

Hips
Insecurity
Poo

Dogs
You Got This!
Sanity
Pets
Lonely
Anguish
Sleep
Insomnia
A light at the end of the tunnel!

About Wendy

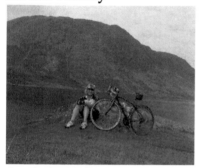

For several years, Wendy knew there was something wrong with her as she repeatedly had groin pain whenever she exercised. No one would believe her until after five years of unnecessary, repeated appointments with various health professionals, when she finally heard her diagnosis of hip dysplasia. It's been tough, but she's a PAO Warrior and proud to have joined such a supportive worldwide group.

Laura Ricci

My PAO Wishbone

You break the bone to get your wish.
They break my pelvis to create new coverage.
Better and stronger than before.

Sometimes with great loss, comes great gain.
Sometimes you have to break down, before you can breakthrough.
You put the pieces together and start anew.

You build a backbone from the wishbone.
These challenges are as much mental, as they are physical.
New beginnings are taking place, a new chapter in my life.

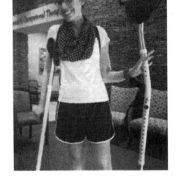

You learn lessons along the way.
This is a time for rest and receiving help.
This is a time for surrender.

In a way, this is a rebirth, a starting over.
Dependent on others like a small child.
Later learning to walk again, taking baby
steps.

You stumble and fall, you get back up.
The process is painful.
Through it, you grow.

One step forward, two steps back.
Recovery is an ever-evolving process.
It requires great strength, patience, and fortitude.

You learn to balance on your new hips.
You find your new equilibrium.
Transformation requires change, and change is not for the faint of
heart.

Your body is now modified, upgraded, and bionic.
You have the scars to prove it.
They are reminders of the miracle that has taken place... you are that miracle.

Your bone was broken, but your wish was granted.
You realize you are stronger than you ever thought possible.
You take that strength with you, as you confidently walk out into the world, on your new hips.

About Laura

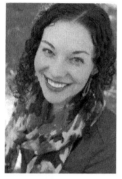

Dr. Laura Ricci is a licensed doctor of physical therapy specializing in Women's Health and Pelvic Floor Rehabilitation, as well as a certified Women's Health Nutrition Coach (WHNC) through the Integrative Women's Health Institute (IWHI). Through her own medical challenges, including cancer and major orthopedic surgery, she found a passion for nutrition. Since Laura had so much personal experience with surgery and recovery, she wrote and taught the Nutrition Pre- and Post-Abdominal and Pelvic Surgery course for the IWHI, due to her extensive experience in both areas.

Laura enjoys learning and expanding her knowledge in the areas of functional medicine and nutrition. She has completed a one-year certification in holistic health coaching and nutrition through the IWHI, and she is currently completing a two-year Nutritional Endocrinology Practitioner Training Program through the Institute of Nutritional Endocrinology.

Laura teaches nutrition classes, cooking classes, and provides private, one-on-one nutrition and health coaching virtually all over the globe: www.lauraricci.vpweb.com.

She strives to be a light in the darkness, offering hope for others with her personal story of love and healing. She lives with her husband in Amarillo, Texas, where she loves healthy cooking, going to Tai Chi class, and spending time in nature.

Jill Campbell

Haiku for PAO Recovery

My socket is flat

My doctor sawed, drilled, and screwed

Soon I'll walk again

About Jill

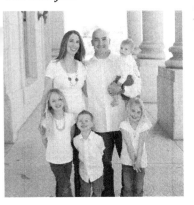

Jill is a 31-year-old mother of four and former (small-time) college soccer player. She and her family live on the central California coast, though they're originally from Salt Lake City. They love to travel and will be living abroad in China soon, so being pain-free is an exciting goal!

Geraldine O'Sullivan

Ode to a Hip

Oh little hip, you've been through so much!
First they signed you, then cut you, then drilled you and such.
With all of that work, it's been quite an ordeal.
But now you can rest and get better and heal!
You won't be able to run outside and get muddy —
But at least you're glued together with bone putty!
With those new crutches you'll be looking quite foxy,
And you'll be feeling no pain thanks to plenty of Oxy!
You might feel like you're moving slow as a sloth,
But soon you'll be back to full strength with bone broth!
When you're off of the meds we'll walk to a bar,
And on Halloween you can show off your new scar!
And so little hip don't forget to stay strong —
You'll be back to yourself before too long!

About Geraldine

Geraldine works as a school social worker providing mental health counseling services to high school students in Escondido, California. When her roommate got diagnosed with hip dysplasia and she saw how difficult the whole process was, she thought it would be nice to write a little poem for her roommate after her surgery to cheer her up. Maybe it can do the same for others!

Glossary and Endnotes

Glossary

5K	Five kilometer (3.1 miles) running road race, which is very popular for recreation.
Acetabular anteversion	A form of acetabular dysplasia resulting in abnormal anterior coverage in the hip joint.[4]
Acetabular retroversion	A form of acetabular dysplasia resulting in abnormal posterior coverage in the hip joint. [4]
Acetametophin	"A drug for pain relief and reduce a fever. It is the active ingredient in Tylenol." [5]
AP X-ray	Anterior pelvic X-ray. An X-ray view that may show hip dysplasia.
Arthrogram	"A test using X-rays to obtain a series of pictures of a joint after a contrast material (such as a dye, water, air, or a combination of these) has been injected into the joint. This allows your doctor to see the soft tissue structures of your joint, such as tendons, ligaments, muscles, cartilage, and your joint capsule. These structures are not seen on a plain X-ray without contrast material. A special type of X-ray, called fluoroscopy, is used to take pictures of the joint.
	"An arthrogram is used to check a joint to find out what is causing your symptoms or problem with your joint. An arthrogram may be more useful than a regular X-ray because it shows the surface of soft tissues lining the joint as well as the joint bones. A regular X-ray only shows the bones of the joint. This test can be done on your hip, knee, ankle, shoulder, elbow, wrist, or jaw (temporomandibular joint).

"Other tests, such as magnetic resonance imaging (MRI) and computed tomography (CT), give different information about a joint. They may be used with an arthrogram or when an arthrogram does not give a clear picture of the joint." [6]

Arthroscopy   "A procedure for diagnosing and treating joint problems." [7]

Bursae   "A small fluid-filled sac or saclike cavity situated in places in tissues where friction would otherwise occur. adj., *adj* bur′sal. Bursae function to facilitate the gliding of muscles or tendons over bony or ligamentous surfaces. They are numerous and are found throughout the body; the most important are located at the shoulder, elbow, knee, and hip." [8]

C-E Angle   Center Edge Angle. A common measurement for the depth of the hip socket. [9]

CNA   Certified Nursing Assistant

Cortisone   A steroid hormone. Cortisone injections may be used to reduce inflammation in a specific area of the body. [10]

CT scan   aka CAT Scan. An image produced by Computerized Axial Tomography. [11]

DDH   Developmental dysplasia of the hip. Commonly referred as: hip dysplasia.

DFO   "Derotational Femoral Osteotomy. **Femoral osteotomy** is a surgical procedure that is performed to correct specific deformities of the femur - the long bone in the upper leg - and the hip joint." [12]

EDS   "Ehlers-Danlos Syndrome. Individuals with Ehlers-Danlos syndromes (EDS) have a genetic defect in their connective tissue, the tissue that provides support to many body parts such as the skin, muscles and ligaments. The fragile skin and unstable joints found in patients with EDS are the result of faulty or reduced amounts of collagen." [13]

FAI   Femoral Acetabular Impingment

Gabapentin   Generic name of Neurontin, a medication that is may be prescribed for treatment of nerve pain.

ICU   Intensive Care Unit. Special care unit in a hospital for life-threatening conditions.

IV   Intravenous; a device that is used to allow a fluid (such as blood or a liquid medication) to flow directly into a patient's veins.[14]

L4-L5   4th and 5th Lumbar vertebrae, bones in the lower spine. It is a common area that is subject to pain due to injury or degenerative changes. [15]

Labral tear   "A hip labral tear involves the ring of cartilage, called the labrum, that follows the outside rim of the socket of your hip joint. The labrum acts like a rubber seal or gasket to help hold the ball at the top of your thighbone securely within your hip socket.

"Athletes who participate in such sports as ice hockey, soccer, football, golfing and ballet are at higher risk of developing a hip labral tear. Structural abnormalities of the hip also can lead to a hip labral tear."[16]

Labrum	"In medicine, a ring of fibrocartilage (fibrous cartilage) around the edge of the articular (joint) surface of a bone. The term labrum is used in anatomy to designate a lip, edge, or brim. Plural: labra."[17]
Lidocaine	"Lidocaine hydrochloride injection, USP is sterile, nonpyrogenic, aqueous solution that contains a local anesthetic agent and is administered parenterally by injection. Lidocaine can also be administered topically in a cream, oil, or patch."[18]
LPAO	Left [hip] Periacetabular Osteotomy. See also: *PAO*
Lyrica	"Also known as Pregabalin, is an anti-epileptic drug, also called an anticonvulsant. It works by slowing down impulses in the brain that cause seizures. Pregabalin also affects chemicals in the brain that send pain signals across the nervous system."[19]
MRI	"Magnetic resonance imaging (MRI) is a test that uses a magnetic field and pulses of radio wave energy to make pictures of organs and structures inside the body. In many cases, MRI gives different information about structures in the body than can be seen with an X-ray, ultrasound, or computed tomography (CT) scan."[20]
MRI Arthrogram	An MRI that follows an arthrogram (contrast dye). See also: *Arthrogram*
Obturator nerve	"The obturator nerve is a large nerve arising from the lumbar plexus and the nerve of the **medial compartment of the thigh.** It arises from the anterior divisions of L2-4 in the **lumbar plexus.**"[21]

Open [hip] dislocation	"Open hip dislocation refers to a surgical procedure in which the ball-and-socket hip joint is surgically dislocated so that the natural hip joint can be repaired. Open hip dislocation can be an extremely effective way to correct complex hip disorders while preserving your natural hip joint."[22]
OR	Operating Room
PACU	Post-Anesthesia Care Unit. Special care unit in a hospital.
PAO	"Periacetabular Osteotomy, or PAO, is a surgical treatment for acetabular dysplasia that preserves and enhances your own hip joint rather than replacing it with an artificial part." [23]
Pavlik cast (harness)	"The Pavlik harness is specially designed to gently position [infants'] hips so they are aligned in the joint, and to keep the hip joint secure. It is typically used to treat babies from birth to six months of age." [24]
PFO	Partial Femoral Osteotomy. See Femoral Osterotomy (FO).
Physio	Another term, often used in Great Britain and Australia, for Physical Therapy.
PICC line	"A peripherally inserted central catheter, or PICC line (say "pick"), is a central venous catheter inserted into a vein in the arm rather than a vein in the neck or chest."[25]
Piriformis	"A muscle that arises from the front of the sacrum, passes out of the pelvis through the greater sciatic foramen, is inserted into the upper border of the

greater trochanter of the femur, and rotates the thigh laterally."[26]

Pleural effusion
"A buildup of fluid in the pleural space, an area between the layers of tissue that line the lungs and the chest cavity. It may also be referred to as effusion or pulmonary effusion." [27]

PM&R
"Physical medicine and rehabilitation (PM&R), also called physiatry, is the branch of medicine emphasizing the prevention, diagnosis, and treatment of disorders – particularly related to the nerves, muscles, and bones – that may produce temporary or permanent impairment." [28]

Prolotherapist
"A person who practices prolotherapy. Prolotherapy is a treatment technique used for chronic myofascial pain, back pain, osteoarthritis, or sports injury. It involves repeated injections of dextrose solution or other irritating substances into the joint, tendon, or painful tissue in order to provoke a regenerative tissue response."[29]

PT
Physical Therapy

RPAO
Right [side] Periacetabular Osteotomy. See also: *PAO*

Sacroiliac/ SI Joint
"The joint formed by the sacrum and ilium where they meet on either side of the lower back. The tight joint allows little motion and is subject to great stress as the body's weight pushes downward and the legs and pelvis push upward against the joint. The sacroiliac joint must also bear the leverage demands made by the trunk of the body as it turns, twists, pulls, and pushes. When these motions place an excess of stress on the ligaments binding the joint

and on the connecting muscles (such as during weightlifting), strain may result." [30]

Spica cast "While the Spica Cast itself is not a surgical procedure, the spica cast is generally used after a surgical procedure for hip dysplasia. This is because the hip joint needs to be kept in the new, surgically repaired hip joint position to ensure proper development of the hip joint."[31]

Sublaxated Partially dislocated. [32]

TFL "Tensor Fasciae Latae muscle. a muscle that arises especially from the anterior part of the iliac crest and from the anterior superior iliac spine, is inserted into the iliotibial band of the fascia lata about one third of the way down the thigh, and acts to flex and abduct the thigh." [33]

THR Total hip replacement.

Torticollis "Also called twisted neck or wryneck, is a condition in which an infant holds his or her head tilted to one side and has difficulty turning the head. The cause of congenital muscular torticollis is unknown, however, it may be related to abnormal positioning (breech position, for example) or "crowding" of the baby while in the uterus. This results in an injury to the neck muscle that scars as it heals. The amount of scar in the muscle determines how tight the muscle is.

"Having tighter space in the uterus is more common for first-born children, who are more likely to have torticollis, as well as hip dysplasia." [34]

Tramadol	"Tramadol is [prescribed] to relieve moderate to moderately severe pain, including pain after surgery. The extended-release or long-acting tablets are used for chronic ongoing pain.
	"Tramadol belongs to the group of medicines called opioid analgesics. It acts in the central nervous system (CNS) to relieve pain. When tramadol is used for a long time, it may become habit-forming (causing mental or physical dependence). Physical dependence may lead to side effects when you stop taking the medicine."[35]
Valium	"Diazepam is [prescribed] to relieve symptoms of anxiety and alcohol withdrawal. This medicine may also be used to treat certain seizure disorders and help relax muscles or relieve muscle spasm.
	"Diazepam is a benzodiazepine. Benzodiazepines belong to the group of medicines called central nervous system (CNS) depressants, which are medicines that slow down the nervous system."[36]
Van Rosen Brace	"A hip abduction brace (aka Van Rosen splint) used to treat hip dysplasia in infants." [37]
Vestibulectomy	"Surgical removal of the vestibule and hymen."[38]

Notes

[1] "World Health Organization Supports Global Effort to Relieve Chronic Pain." *World Health Organization*, 11 Oct. 2004. Web. 1 Nov. 2015. <http://www.who.int/mediacentre/news/releases/2004/pr70/en>.

[2] "What is Hip Dysplasia?" International Hip Dysplasia Institute, 2012. Web. 5 Nov. 2015. <http://hipdysplasia.org>.

[3] Eponis | Synope. "Everything Is Awful, and I'm Not Okay: Questions to Ask Before Giving Up." Tumblr. Web. 26 Oct. 2015. <http://eponis.tumblr.com/post/113798088670/everything-is-awful-and-im-not-okay-questions-to>.

[4] "Femoral Version: Definition, Diagnosis, and Intraoperative Correction With Modular Femoral Components." *Healio*. 1 Sept. 2005. Web. 5 Nov. 2015. <http://www.healio.com/orthopedics/hip/news/online>.

[5] "Acetaminophen." *Drugs.com*. 2015. Web. 6 Nov. 2015. <http://www.drugs.com/acetaminophen.html>.

[6] "Arthrogram (Joint X-Ray)." *WebMD*. WebMD Medical Reference from Healthwise, 9 Sept. 2014. Web. 5 Nov. 2015. <http://www.webmd.com/arthritis/arthrogram-joint-x-ray>.

[7] "Tests and Procedures: Arthroscopy." *Mayo Clinic*. Mayo Clinic Staff, 17 June 2015. Web. 7 Nov. 2015. <http://www.mayoclinic.org/tests-procedures/arthroscopy/basics/definition/prc-20014669?reDate=28112015>.

[8] "Bursae." *The Free Dictionary*. Farlex, Inc., 2015. Web. 6 Nov. 2015. <http://medical-dictionary.thefreedictionary.com/bursae>.

[9] "Adult Diagnosis." *International Hip Dysplasia Institute*. 2012. Web. 7 Nov. 2015. <http://hipdysplasia.org/adult-hip-dysplasia/adult-diagnosis>.

[10] "Tests and Procedures: Cortisone Shots." *Mayo Clinic*. Mayo Clinic Staff, 13 Aug. 2013. Web. 7 Nov. 2015. <http://www.mayoclinic.org/tests-procedures/cortisone-shots/basics/definition/prc-20014455>.

[11] "CT Scan." *The Free Dictionary*. Farlex, Inc., 2015. Web. 6 Nov. 2015. <http://medical-dictionary.thefreedictionary.com/CT+scan>.

[12] Buly, Robert L. "Femoral Osteotomy." *Hospital for Special Surgery*. 1 Jan. 2015. Web. 6 Nov. 2015. <https://www.hss.edu/conditions_femoral-osteotomy-overview.asp>.

[13] "What Is EDS?" *EDNF*. Ehlers-Danlos National Foundation, 2015. Web. 6 Nov. 2015. <http://ednf.org/what-eds>.

[14] "IV." *Merriam-Webster Dictionary*. Merriam-Webster, Incorporated, 2015. Web. 5 Nov. 2015. <http://www.merriam-webster.com/dictionary/iv>.

[15] DeWitt, David. "All about the L4-L5 Spinal Segment." *Spine-Health: Trusted Information for Back Pain*. 29 Oct. 2013. Web. 6 Nov. 2015. <http://www.spine-health.com/conditions/spine-anatomy/all-about-l4-l5-spinal-segment>.

[16] "Diseases and Conditions: Hip Labral Tear." *Mayo Clinic*. Mayo Clinic Staff, 23 Apr. 2015. Web. 7 Nov. 2015. <http://www.mayoclinic.org/diseases-conditions/hip-labral-tear/basics/definition/con-20031062>.

[17] "Definition of Labrum." *MedicineNet*. MedicineNet. Inc., 14 June 2012. Web. 5 Nov. 2015. <http://www.medicinenet.com/script/main/art.asp?articlekey=18656>.

[18] "Lidocaine." *Drugs.com*. Dec. 2014. Web. 6 Nov. 2015. <http://www.drugs.com/pro/lidocaine.html>.

[19] "Lyrica." *RxList: The Internet Drug Index*. RxList, Inc., 2015. Web. 5 Nov. 2015. <http://www.rxlist.com/lyrica-drug/patient-images-side-effects.htm>.

[20] "Magnetic Resonance Imaging (MRI)." *WebMD*. WebMD, LLC, 9 Sept. 2014. Web. 7 Nov. 2015. <http://www.webmd.com/a-to-z-guides/magnetic-resonance-imaging-mri>.

[21] Hacking, Craig, and Aaron Wong, et al. "Obturator Nerve." *Radiopaedia.org*. 2015. Web. 6 Nov. 2015. <http://radiopaedia.org/articles/obturator-nerve>.

[22] Clohisy, John. "Treatment Options: Open Hip Dislocation." *John Clohisy, MD*. n.d. Web. 7 Nov. 2015. <http://www.clohisyhipsurgeon.com/treatment-options/open-hip-dislocation>.

[23] Sink, Ernest L. "Periacetabular Osteotomy (PAO)." *Hospital for Special Surgery*. n.d. Web. 5 Nov. 2015. <https://www.hss.edu/physician-files/sink/SinkPAO5.8.12.pdf>.

[24] "Infant and Child Hip Dysplasia: Pavlik Harness." *International Hip Dysplasia Institute*. 2012. Web. 6 Nov. 2015. <http://hipdysplasia.org/developmental-dysplasia-of-the-hip/child-treatment-methods/pavlik-harness/ #sthash. qJ9mwTd2.dpuf>.

[25] "Pain Management Health Center: Central Venous Catheters - Topic Overview." *WebMD*. WebMD Medical Reference from Healthwise, 14 Nov. 2014. Web. 6 Nov. 2015. <http://www.webmd.com/pain-management/tc/central-venous-catheters-topic-overview>.

[26] "Piriformis." *Merriam-Webster Medical Dictionary*. Merriam-Webster, Incorporated, 2015. Web. 5 Nov. 2015. <http://www.merriam-webster.com/ medical/piriformis>.

[27] Davis, Charles Patrick. "Pleural Effusion (Fluid In the Chest or On the Lung)." *MedicineNet.com*. MedicineNet, Inc., 6 Feb. 2015. Web. 5 Nov. 2015. <http://www.medicinenet.com/ pleural_effusion_fluid_in_the_chest_or_on_lung/article.htm>.

[28] "Patients and Family: FAQs about PM&R." *AAPM&R*. American Academy of Physical Medicine and Rehabilitation, 2015. Web. 5 Nov. 2015. <https://www.aapmr.org/patients/aboutpmr/ Pages/FAQs.aspx>.

[29] Novella, Steven. "Prolotherapy." *Science-Based Medicine*. 11 June 2014. Web. 5 Nov. 2015. <https://www.sciencebasedmedicine.org/ prolotherapy>.

[30] "Sacroiliac Joint." *The Free Dictionary*. Farlex, Inc., 2015. Web. 6 Nov. 2015. <http://medical-dictionary.thefreedictionary.com/ sacroiliac+joint>.

[31] "Infant and Child Hip Dysplasia: Hip Spica Cast." *International Hip Dysplasia Institute*. 2012. Web. 6 Nov. 2015. <http://hipdysplasia.org/developmental-dysplasia-of-the-hip/child-treatment-methods/hip-spica-cast>.

[32] "Subluxated." *Merriam-Webster Medical Dictionary*. Merriam-Webster, Incorporated, 2015. Web. 5 Nov. 2015. <http://www.merriam-webster.com/medical/subluxated>.

[33] "Tensor Fasciae Latae." *Merriam-Webster Medical Dictionary*. Merriam-Webster, Incorporated, 2015. Web. 5 Nov. 2015. <http://www.merriam-webster.com/medical/tensor fasciae latae>.

34 "Congenital Muscular Torticollis (Twisted Neck)." *OrthoInfo*. American Academy of Orthopaedic Surgeons, Mar. 2013. Web. 7 Nov. 2015. <http://orthoinfo.aaos.org/topic.cfm?topic=a00054>.

35 "Drugs and Supplements: Tramadol (Oral Route)." *Mayo Clinic*. Micromedex, 1 Nov. 2015. Web. 5 Nov. 2015. <http://www.mayoclinic.org/drugs-supplements/tramadol-oral-route/description/drg-20068050>.

36 "Drugs and Supplements: Diazepam (Oral Route)." *Mayo Clinic*. Micromedex, 1 Nov. 2015. Web. 5 Nov. 2015. <http://www.mayoclinic.org/drugs-supplements/diazepam-oral-route/description/drg-20072333>.

37 "Infant and Child Hip Dysplasia: Von Rosen Splint." *International Hip Dysplasia Institute*. 2012. Web. 6 Nov. 2015. <http://hipdysplasia.org/developmental-dysplasia-of-the-hip/child-treatment-methods/von-rosen-splint>.

38 "Vestibulectomy." *The Free Dictionary*. Farlex, Inc., 2015. Web. 6 Nov. 2015. <http://medical-dictionary.thefreedictionary.com/Vestibulectomy>.

About *The PAO Project*™

There is little information about adult hip dysplasia and the hip preservation surgery, Periacetabular Osteotomy (PAO), especially from a patient's perspective. In fact, when searching online for "hip dysplasia," there is more information about *canine* hip dysplasia vs. *human* hip dysplasia!

While blogs and support groups exist online, Jennifer Lesea-Ames was inspired through her own experience of being diagnosed with bilateral hip dysplasia at the age of 39 and undergoing PAO surgery in April 2014 and December 2014 to start *The PAO Project*™. This project offers an opportunity for those who have been diagnosed with hip dysplasia and have had PAO surgery can submit their heartfelt, soul journey stories for consideration to be published in the anthology, *Onward: Navigating through Hip Dysplasia, PAO Surgery, and Beyond, Volume 1.*

With your donations, Jennifer Lesea-Ames can continue to maintain *The PAO Project*™ website and provide support services and financial assistance for PAO warriors. For example, a long-term goal of The PAO Project™ is to use these donations to provide micro-grants to help those diagnosed with hip dysplasia and PAO patients pay for surgery recovery equipment, or pay the shipping to swap equipment among patients.

Want to learn more about this project?

Interested in making a donation to the project?

Visit http://ThePAOProject.com

Made in the USA
San Bernardino, CA
25 February 2018